Praise for
Stop Calling Him Honey and Start Having Sex

"I'm not sure if familiarity breeds contempt in marriage, but I'm sure
it breed‹   ⟩ in a
sexual r   con-
crete ad   met.
Their ‹   the
sexual s

—   *iage,*
                                                          sting

"What   ong-
term re   rom
the gut,   rev-
olutioni   rant
fun-lovi

                                                       sire:
                                                       sion
                                                       Sex

"I love   get
press, bu   dif-
ferentia   sys-
tems. I

                                                        my
                                                       t of
                                                       t It

stop calling him
Honey...
and start having
Sex!

How Changing Your Everyday
Habits Will Make You *Hot* for
Each Other All Over Again

Maggie Arana and Julienne Davis

Health Communications, Inc.
Deerfield Beach, Florida

Library of Congress Cataloging-in-Publication Data

Arana, Maggie.
    Stop calling him "honey"—and start having sex! : how changing your everyday habits will make you hot for each other all over again / Maggie Arana and Julienne Davis.
        p. cm.
    Includes index.
    ISBN-13: 978-0-7573-1531-2
    ISBN-10: 0-7573-1531-3
    1. Sex instruction.   2. Man-woman relationships.   3. Sex counseling.
    I. Davis, Julienne.   II. Title.
    HQ56.A7378 2010
    646.7'8—dc22

                                                        2010011515

Publisher: Health Communications, Inc.
        3201 S.W. 15th Street
        Deerfield Beach, FL 33442–8190

Cover photos ©iStockphoto, ©newphotoservice
Interior design and formatting by Lawna Patterson Oldfield

To the memory of my mother, Mary Arana,
who I wish could be a young woman today
and enjoy the opportunity to live a joyous
and self-fulfilling life.

—Maggie Arana

To Jay, my wonderful husband
and the love of my life.

—Julienne Davis

Contents

Acknowledgments

TO JAY STRONGMAN—for being our first advocate and our first editor. Thanks for helping to turn our writing (especially the early stuff) into something that resembles the English language. Thanks for improving our cadence and our "clunkers"—and no, you don't have to leave the room!

To Norm Kerner—for your love, input, and support . . . and your patience for putting up with many days and nights without Maggie while we were writing this book.

To Sannah Wheatley—for your love, your support, and your wonderful friendship.

To Laurie Abkemeier—for being such an amazing agent, and always keeping us informed and up-to-date. Thanks for believing in us and for your fabulous input on how to make our book even better. When you said in our first phone conversation, "If you're on board, I'm on board," we knew we'd found the best agent that two girls could ever ask for.

To Michele Matrisciani and all at HCI Books—for your excitement, enthusiasm, and belief in our book.

To all of our friends, acquaintances, and even strangers—for allowing us a glimpse into the most intimate and personal part of your lives and loves. Without all of you, we could have never written this book.

Preface:
Why We Had to Write This Book

REMEMBER WHEN YOU WERE young and all you could think about with your new lover was when you were going to have sex? You'd plan it, dream about it, and pretty much do whatever you had to do to get it. You were ready and raring to go, right? So, what's happened with that? Why did all that change? Now that you don't have to sneak around high school to find a secluded corner to make out or eagerly await the next school dance (where it was really *dark*), what the hell happened? After all, you are still young at heart, and you can do it as much as you want to now . . . and yet, you don't. And when it gets to the point where you are asking each other, "Let's see, shall we have sex or watch another *Seinfeld* rerun?" you know it's time to seek some answers before all your sexual bits just shrivel up!

We came to realize that in our own lives and those of other couples, too, this issue needed some serious attention. But first, we felt we needed to find out why this happens to couples to begin with, and then, by knowing the cause of the problem, we'd hopefully find a solution. We wanted to feel the way we did when we were young—wouldn't you? Now, we're pretty sure that many of you picked up the book, read the title, and thought, "What the hell does *that* mean?" Well, read on, and we'll explain.

We never thought we'd be writing a self-help sex book. Ten years ago, it wouldn't have even occurred to us to even write a book, let alone one on sex in long-term relationships! But here we are. In our own lives, we found ourselves in that familiar situation that a lot of couples fall into when they've been together for a few years: you love each other, you may even consider each other best friends, but the sex is not like it was in the beginning. If you're doing it at all, that is.

We're not therapists and we don't pretend to be, but the expert advice we each read on the subject didn't do a thing for us. Sure, there have been numerous books and articles written by traditional therapists and so-called experts, which sound like good advice, with suggestions for "how to spice up your sex life," including, ad nauseam, all the usual things you should do to jump-start your sexual selves again: communicating your "intimacy needs" to your partner, wearing sexy lingerie, having a date night, role playing, sex toys, and even having sex in places like on the kitchen table or in the neighbor's yard! In fact, some even suggest "forcing yourself" to "just do it anyway"—thinking this will increase your desire to have more sex. Guess what? It doesn't! Forcing yourself to do something you just don't want to do is going to make you feel stupid at best—and, at worst, resentful toward your partner. You may even become annoyed at yourself because you feel like you *should* want to "just do it." But you don't. Desire is something you just can't fake. And, many of you have probably tried some or all of these "sexual spicer-uppers," that the "experts" advise, but in the end we're guessing they changed nothing. Why? We asked the same question, and we were determined to seek our own answers to this common dilemma.

This is not a book that developed overnight, but one that has come from almost ten years of the two of us searching and finally finding what really works to keep a couple's sex life hot.

How We Met

From the moment we met, we knew we would be good friends. As our friendship grew, we realized how much we related to one another on many levels. Throughout most of our adult lives, neither one of us liked the idea of flitting from one relationship to another because we both valued long-term commitment. When we began talking about the dilemma of keeping sex hot after many years with the same person, writing this book became necessary for us—not only for ourselves in our own relationships, but for others, too. And even though we were novice writers, it was a surprisingly easy process because so much of our book is from actual people simply being truthful with us, as well as us being truthful with ourselves and with each other.

Julienne recalls:

"Maggie and I first met through a mutual English friend in Los Angeles in 1997. We instantly hit it off because we had a lot in common. Sharing a strong interest in retro fashion, music, and midcentury homes, we became fast friends (along with our respective partners), even though my husband and I were still living in London, while Maggie and her boyfriend resided in Los Angeles. Because of my acting career (and the fabulous weather), my husband and I visited L.A. several times a year, and it was always a highlight of those trips for the four of us to get together. We all went together to the L.A. premiere of Stanley Kubrick's *Eyes Wide Shut*, a film in which I had a pivotal role. The film, starring Tom Cruise and Nicole Kidman, explored the dynamic between marital fidelity and sexual desire.

"Looking back, I think it was the content of that film that really started Maggie and me thinking about sexual fulfillment in our own respective relationships. We had many private conversations about our sexual pasts—the good, the bad, and definitely the ugly! We had both experienced lack of desire in our long-term relationships, and we were perplexed as to why this always seems to happen, even when the partnership can be great on so many other levels. Time passed, and by 2005, my husband and I were considering a permanent move to Los Angeles. While checking our work prospects, I ended up spending several months living, on and off, with Maggie. She had recently broken up with her partner of twenty years, and she welcomed the company.

"As close girlfriends tend to do, we spent many evenings talking about what had gone wrong in Maggie's seemingly strong relationship and how the lack of sex played a part in its demise. We both tried to understand why a couple's sex life tends to suffer after the first few years and why this *always* seems to happen. More particularly, we asked ourselves, why did Maggie's relationship end up being sexually barren when she and her boyfriend had such a great partnership, had so much in common, and enjoyed spending most of their time together? Everyone we knew thought they were a great couple. They did everything together and seemed very, very close. Whenever we saw them together, they seemed like the *last* couple in the room that you'd ever suspect to have problems. Earlier in our friendship, it was sometimes even difficult for me to talk to Maggie on her own because she and her partner seemed so engaged with each other. They were like a singular unit—two halves of a whole."

Maggie continues:

"It was during this time that Julienne and I had an epiphany: it seemed that no matter how strong the partnership or how deep the friendship, if couples fell into certain bad habits, their sex lives suffered. Looking back, I realized that my own sex life started to disappear when my partner and I began using pet names and baby talk with each other. Likewise, when we discussed Julienne's past relationships, she realized that her own sex life had suffered for the same reasons as mine. We both found that we used names like 'honey,' 'sweetie,' and 'pookie,' and were generally much too comfortable with our partners. This led to our realization that *honey* is a very dangerous word and leads to further bad habits that can ultimately destroy the sexual chemistry between partners, and even the relationship itself, if left unchecked. My partner and I probably did seem like the perfect couple because we truly did love each other's company. There was no one with whom I'd rather talk with than him, and I think he felt the same about me. At home, however, we had so many bad habits going on that feeling sexual with each other was virtually impossible. And I think that's the main reason our relationship ended—because no matter how strong the friendship or how deep the bond, a love relationship needs to have sexual intimacy to survive."

After this discovery, we set out to find if this often happened in other people's relationships. Over the last several years, we've talked to many friends and acquaintances currently in long-term relationships. To our surprise, we found that nearly *all* of them suffered from humdrum sex lives! These same women and men also admitted to commonly using "honey" and other pet names with their partners. We also got the same "honey" comments when we took our theory a step further and talked to other family members, coworkers, and even people on the Internet. After further inquiry, they also told us that they had more sex before pet names became a daily occurrence. Many women said they couldn't even remember the last time their partner called them by their proper name.

People also revealed how they began to do "everything" in front of their partners within the first year or so of their relationships. This hit home with us as well because we realized we were guilty of the same things in our past relationships. Like our friends and acquaintances, we had never made the connection between these bad habits and a lack of sex. Just like the people we talked to, we realized that some of the habits we used at home probably didn't help our sex lives, but we never thought to change these behaviors because we didn't think they were that important. We had read some of those self-help sex books, but since they didn't say anything about these behaviors damaging our sex lives, we didn't make any changes in these areas. And guess what? No change occurred in our sex lives either! Until we tried the "honey" theories, that is.

Our next step was to read as many books on the subject as we could find, thinking that at least *one* therapist must have made the same connection we had. We were shocked to find out that *none* of the therapists had made the "honey" connection. Also, none of them mentioned the further connection between our everyday habits and the inadvertent sabotage of our sex lives. No one addressed these obvious causes, but to us, it seemed clear—it was the elephant in the room!

So, from our own experiences and from several years of talking to hundreds of men and women, we discovered the actual cause of a fading sex life. The books we had read were focused on merely treating the symptoms, like putting a Band-Aid on an infected wound, while the advice in our book treats the infection itself.

We also found that most of the other books we read on the subject were extremely academic, and because of this, they offered very little in the way of effective and understandable advice. The therapists' opinions might have made sense for an academic paper, but they didn't really work in the average couple's day-to-day life. Even though we consider ourselves to be fairly intelligent women, most of the self-help books we found on the shelves were so cerebral that they were pretty much unreadable; explanations of "how the neocortex part of your brain effects your libido" weren't really helpful. (We didn't care what part of our brain controlled sexual desire; we just wanted to have more sex with our partners again!) We concluded that real and practical help for the average woman was sadly missing and sorely needed. We wanted to change that. We wanted to write a book that women (and men) would want to read—the truth, straight up, with no "therapy-speak"—based on real experience and what actually works, whether you're in a long-term relationship or just starting out in one.

Our book is not just about a single word, however. That's only the first step in the process. The first three chapters in this book focus on what you need to *stop* doing to let a natural sexual chemistry happen again, and the chapters after that explain what to *start* doing. We found that after we and many others tried the techniques we illustrate in our book, invigorating our sex lives wasn't hard work at all—that's just another myth most of us have been led to believe. These are easy changes that lead to a natural desire to have sex, something we know we have all missed in our relationships.

So Here's What You Need to Ask Yourself . . .

You and your significant other have been together for a while now, right? You're in a great relationship. You're communicating. There's a lot of "spooning" going on. You probably consider each other best friends. You have a very good partnership. But . . . are you actually having great sex?

And by that we mean the hot, frantic kind of sex that you had when you first got together. The kind of sex where you look into each other's eyes and want to rip each other's clothes off. The kind of sex where you can't even wait to get to the bedroom and end up doing it on the stairs. The kind of sex that has you wet with anticipation. No? We didn't think so.

We both know that even when the companionship is great and you and your partner love each other deeply, eventually you'll find something missing in the bedroom. And sometimes, that little something can eat away at what once was a great relationship. Sex can become ho-hum or humdrum . . . and at that point, then what?

Two possibilities: celibacy or cheating. One or the other. But it doesn't have to be that way!

The sad thing about what happens to sexless relationships is that one partner will eventually cheat—not with a person who is any better than his or her current partner, but with someone who relates and communicates the way you both used to.

At this point in your life you might even be thinking, *But I'm just not that interested in sex. I've been there, done that, many times before. I just don't need it or crave it anymore.* But a love relationship without sex or physical intimacy takes its toll on the partnership, no matter how strong you think your bond might be. And you need to ask yourself: did you really sign up for having just a roommate?

We have discovered that by changing simple, everyday habits, you can stop sabotaging your sex life on a daily basis. You can unlock the passion you had in the beginning and go from being roommates back to the passionate couple you were meant to be. That is the reason we felt we had to write this book: to share this groundbreaking advice with all of those couples out there who are getting a little bored with their sex life and are starting to head down that slippery slope of celibacy or cheating. Don't we all wax lyrical about those early days? Imagine how invigorated, young, and vibrant you would feel if you could get just a little of that feeling back again. We know, we're excited too, so read on, and let's stop calling him "honey" and start having sex again!

Introduction: A Brief History of Honey

WHERE DID THE USE OF THE WORD *HONEY* as a term of endearment come from? Of all the words available, why is this the word we have all called each other for hundreds of years? And why is it still being used? How did nicknames between couples come about anyway? And why are they so common? Did Adam say to Eve, "Oh, honey . . . please don't eat that apple!" Well, we did some research and here's what we found.

As a basic word, *honey* was originally derived from the old English word *hunig*. This first usage of *honey* with its current spelling is documented in the Oxford English Dictionary as occurring in the year 875. Back then, as it is today, its meaning was for that yummy sweet stuff we like to put on toast. As terms of endearment, the use of the words *honey* and *sweetheart* can be traced back to as early as the 1300s. They are the oldest and still most common words that couples use to address each other.

Interestingly enough, besides the obvious meaning of *sweet*, honey was once considered a valuable commodity. In some cases, the Romans even used honey instead of gold as a form of payment for taxes. The ancient Egyptians also saw honey as a symbol of fertility, and it was used as an offering to Min, the Fertility God. And in Hinduism, honey (*Madhu*) is one of the five elixirs of immortality.

One of the first known written examples of *honey* and *sweetheart* appearing as terms of endearment was in Geoffrey Chaucer's *Canterbury Tales*; namely, "The Miller's Tale" (circa 1380). A miller in medieval times was a man who ground grain into flour—a very common working-class profession at the time; hence the common surname today of Miller. This first "honey" was an eighteen-year old woman named Alison who was married to a much older man who was a carpenter by trade. In the common medieval tale of a cuckolded husband, Alison is sleeping with a young student who rents a room in their home, while also flirting with a dandy (a well-dressed and/or vain gentleman) who calls on her from time to time. The student convinces the not-so-bright carpenter husband that there might be a flood coming and that he should build a boat to save them. The husband is so distracted while building the boat that the sly student now has plenty of time to have sex with the beautiful, young Alison. The following passage from "The Miller's Tale" shows one of the first known instances of the word *honey* being used as a term of endearment:

> *This silly carpenter begins to quake:*
> *He thinketh verily that he may see*
> *This newe flood come weltering as the sea*
> *To drenchen Alison, his honey dear.*

The following is one of the first examples of *sweetheart*, also from "The Miller's Tale":

And secretly he [the student] caught hold of her genitalia and said:
"Surely, unless you will love me, sweetheart, I shall die for my secret
* love of you."*

(Gosh, those medieval guys were awfully forward!)

So, our first known "honey" was a young wife who cheated on her husband with not one, but two other men! Not a very good beginning for the supposed lovey-dovey terms *honey* and *sweetheart*. It seems as if *honey* and *sweetheart* were originally used as cynical, mocking words for a woman who was more slutty than sweet.

Fast forward two hundred years and *honey* appears again, this time in William Shakespeare's *The Taming of the Shrew*, written in 1590. The plot concerns two sisters—the pretty and gentle Bianca and the headstrong Katherina, the shrew. A gentleman named Petruchio pursues and marries Katherina, not for love, but for her father's money as he bluntly states in this passage:

"Kate, eat apace. And now, my honey love,
Will return to her father's house
And revel in it as bravely as the best,
With silken coats and caps and golden rings."

Petruchio wasn't satisfied with just taking his wife's money; he had to have her spirit, too. The play ends with Petruchio "taming" Katherina, and she gives a speech on how women need to obey their husbands. It's obviously a backward view of women when looked at from our modern perspective, but a literary masterpiece nonetheless.

In Shakepeare's *Othello*, written in 1604, *honey* makes another appearance. In this famous tragedy, Othello is a respected general in the Venetian army and married to the beautiful and faithful Desdemona. He says the following to her about his proposed move to Turkey:

> "Honey, you shall be well desir'd in Cyprus,
> I have found great love amongst them."

Unfortunately, many of Othello's officers are plotting against him. At one point, he thinks Desdemona is among the conspirators and he returns to the castle and smothers her to death. Othello then learns that his wife was innocent and kills himself in grief. *Othello* is one of the first known examples where *honey* is used sincerely as a term of endearment. Othello and Desdemona really did love each other, even though he erroneously thought she was a traitor and murdered her as a result.

Compared with *honey* and *sweetheart*, other forms of terms of endearment are relatively recent. The word *baby* as a term of endearment came about much later, in 1839. In the 1800s, the most common nickname between spouses was *dear*, which was first used as early as 1694. *Darling* was first used in the 1500s, and *sugar* started in the 1930s. But none of these words are as old and resilient as our dear old *honey*, which still survives after over six hundred years!

In the 1950s, *honey* was brought into our homes on a regular basis with the advent of television. Remember when Ward Cleaver would come home on *Leave It to Beaver*, when Ozzie Nelson would walk in the door on *The Adventures of Ozzie and Harriet*, or when Jim Anderson would come home on *Father Knows Best*? We definitely heard the phrase *Hi, honey, I'm home!* used a lot.

And from television, America got many of its ideas on how a family should look and behave with each other. Yes, those shows were great, but many of the messages on how a couple should relate to each other probably affected our psyche in not such a great way. In these early shows, husbands and wives called each other "honey" and generally acted in a very nonsexual way. Because of television rules at the time, couples were portrayed sleeping in separate twin beds, and you generally didn't get the feeling that anything sexual would ever happen between them. The wife was often portrayed as a very attractive maid, usually wearing an apron, but always wearing lipstick and having perfectly coiffed hair. Remember June Cleaver? She always looked perfect, even when vacuuming or dusting!

Now we know that some of you may be thinking, *But it's not the fifties anymore, and I don't even remember these shows.* However, the point we're making here is that the use of *honey* in our daily lives and the image of the seemingly platonic married couple have been bombarding us on television for decades. More recently, there was a sitcom in the nineties called *Hi Honey, I'm Home.* Around the same time, there were the hugely popular movies *Honey, I Shrunk the Kids* and the sequel, *Honey, I Blew Up the Kid.*

So, suffice to say, the term of endearment *honey* has been around for a very, very long time. But interestingly, the connotation of this word has often been patronizing or has signified a platonic relationship (as in the case of early television). It's also been bitingly sarcastic (as in our first "honey dear" Allison) or just plain comical (as in *Honey, I Shrunk/Blew Up the Kid(s)*.) Sadly, nowadays, it is so overused that it has become much more of a cliché than a term of endearment. Tired old "honey" has been used for over six hundred years—isn't it time to give it a rest?

Chapter One

Stop Calling Him "Honey"

"I find that the most intimate thing my boyfriend can call me is my name."

—SHARI, AGE 30

"My sweetie and I never call each other by our names unless we're mad at each other. We don't have much sex anymore, but we still love to cuddle."

—AIMEE, AGE 38

IT'S SEEMINGLY ONE OF THE most innocuous words in the world, but for a relationship it can be one of the most dangerous. The word is *honey*. How many of us call our partners "honey"? Millions of us use the word in multiple countries and in multiple languages. Its use has become such a cliché that when we see a film or TV program where a husband returns home from work, we expect to hear him say, "Hi, honey, I'm home!" This is probably one of the most common, socially accepted habits that can develop in long-term relationships. Nearly everyone calls their loved one an endearing nickname. They can't all be wrong can they? Yes, they can! And yes, they are!

What's wrong with calling each other "honey," you ask? Well, honey is great on a warm piece of toast, but lousy on a couple's sex life. Calling your partner "honey" is the first step down the slippery slope toward a bland or nonexistent sexual relationship. And unfortunately, it usually doesn't stop with "honey," but degenerates into "hon," "sweetie," "pookie," "papa bear," "pumpkin," "mugwump," "snookie-ookums," "furfy," "tweetie," "love bug," "cuddle face," "cutie pie," "biscuit," "tiger-twinkies," "doober," "schwinkie," "toodle-puss," "schmoopie". . . you get the picture. And, yes, we could easily fill this entire chapter with the little endearing nicknames that we are all guilty of using. There's a *lot* of creativity goin' on there . . . and that's not helping either!

When you get married, part of the ritual is that you both become one, and that is one of the beautiful things about marriage. You have a permanent partner, an ally, a most-trusted friend. You trust your life, your savings, and most important, your heart with this person. They are your family now. But we need to look further into what "becoming one" actually means.

Once you become one—as in two halves of a whole, rather than two whole complete separate people—you can say good-bye to the passionate sex you enjoyed in the beginning. Why? Because sexual attraction is often built upon being attracted to someone who is different than and separate from you. In marriage, however, this idea of two whole separate people often falls by the wayside after a few years of living together. It's often so easy to get too comfortable with one another and so close that you blur the lines between you and throw part of your identity away in the process. Separation and unique identities are essential to maintaining a good sex life. Becoming one means two whole complete separate people are joined together in marriage. Meaning . . . it's a partnership! It is not that each person gives up half of who they are for that partnership.

The Power in a Name

One of the most important parts of our unique identity is our name. Maybe you have a beautiful name or maybe you have a name that suits your personality. Perhaps your name is the name of a beloved mother or grandmother. Why would you want to lose that? Whether we like it or not, our name is the most obvious sign of our identity. And, it's having a separate identity that makes *any* relationship interesting, whether it's your partner or a friend.

Remember when you first dated your husband—didn't you call him by his name? Sure you did, but how often have you done that lately? We've met many couples in our research for this book that haven't called each other by their real names in years. Many women we talked to said they couldn't even remember the last time their partner said their name to them, and when they did, they usually said something like, "Yeah, now that I think of it, I really miss him calling me by my name at home." What seems to happen is that social mores take over, and we all fall into the same trap of using that age-old endearing nickname: *honey.*

Why is it that you can have a close friend for many years, someone you might speak to every day and share intimate parts of your life with, yet you never resorted to calling that person "honey?" And why do we feel the need to forgo our partner's name just because we are having sex? When we become romantically involved with someone, his or her name usually goes out the window in the first few months and hardly ever returns. One of the most dangerous facets of calling each other "honey" is that it puts your mind in a nonsexual place throughout the day. Then in the evenings or whenever a sexual moment may arise, it is very difficult to get out of the "honey" mind-set.

When you're both calling each other "honey," a small part of your identity is being eroded. Once that happens, you have started down the road to a sexual desert. The power of that seemingly harmless, simple word is amazing. By using it, you inadvertently take the sexual tension down a notch or two in your communication with your lover. Left unchecked, this effectively takes away their individuality, their sex, their female/maleness, and most important, their differentness from you! "Honey" and the like are saccharine sweet, androgynous words. Do you really want to turn your man into a sexless eunuch? Each time you continue to call each other "honey" or some other cute pet name, you chip away at the fact that you are two whole, separate sexual people. You then become two halves of a whole and, contrary to conventional belief, this is not a good thing. Who has sexual tension with the other half of themselves? No one!

You also have to remember that your husband probably has a past, including former girlfriends or wives. Don't you think he called them "honey," too? Why are you okay becoming the latest "honey" in his life? Aren't you better than that? Why would either of you want to be relegated to a generic name? It goes both ways too: if you had past boyfriends where the relationship didn't last, why would you want to fall into the same habits you used before?

Why Turn Down the Flame?

Now you may ask, "But isn't calling him 'honey' just a term of endearment? Doesn't it mean that he's special?" No, it's a term of sameness and nonsexuality. Don't you sometimes call your kids "honey"? Don't you sometimes call your dog or cat "honey?" So, why would you want to call your sexual partner the same thing that you call your six-year-old daughter or your pet poodle? *Honey* has no sexual connotation and no gender. This is not a word you want to use for that man waiting in your bedroom. We're sure many of you out there are thinking, *But we call each other "honey," and we're doing just fine. This just doesn't apply to us.* Well, you may be doing "fine" now, but give it some time, and sure enough, you will be looking back on your nearly sexless relationship and thinking, *What the hell happened to us?* Take heed. *Honey* may seem harmless, but it most definitely is not!

When you start to call each other "honey," you have started to lower the flame on your sex life in many hidden ways. Is that something you want to risk? What good can come of it? Another negative aspect of the word *honey* is that it has a caregiver connotation. That's why your mother and father probably called you "honey" when you were a child—they were taking care of you. That's why you probably sometimes call your child "honey" and why you may call your pet "honey," too—you are taking care of them. But do you really want to call your partner, the one person in your life who is supposed to be your true equal, a word that should really be reserved for someone with whom you have a caregiving role? "Caregiver sex" is never going to be hot sex.

When you were growing up, your parents probably called you "honey" so often that when they actually called you by your real name, you thought you were in trouble. How many of us used to hear from our parents something like, "Mary, come in here, I need to talk to you"? And you quaked in your shoes because you knew your mother or father was angry about something. Unfortunately, what happens between couples is strikingly similar. When we hear our name from our partner (instead of something like "honey-bunny") we probably think, *Uh-oh, I bet he's mad at me.* Being called by your real name has degenerated into such a negative thing, we think our partner is angry with us when it happens! Now how silly is that? Your partner's name is not something to be used solely when you are angry with them. You're not living in your parent's home anymore. You're an adult now, remember? Why prematurely lower the temperature on your sex life with ingrained habits we learned growing up? Is this going to make us hot for one another? Hardly.

Your sex life with your partner is like a campfire. You meet, you both feel those incredible sparks when you're together, and before you know it, you are both feeling the warmth of those flames. But just like a real campfire, your sex life is also subject to outside elements and can easily be put out without you even realizing it. That's why you have to protect your sex life; it won't burn continuously if you allow bad habits to constantly rain on its flame. Every time you allow your communication to devolve into "honey" this and "sweetie" that, you are raining on your sexual campfire. And before long, it's no longer a raging flame, if it's going at all.

Once you've given in to the social custom of forgoing your husband's name for "honey," you have started to desexualize your relationship with him. You are inadvertently turning him into a cuddly teddy-bear friend. "Honey" will bring you a warm cup of cocoa, but "honey" is not going to fuck you. "Honey" is great at spooning under the covers, but not so great for hot passionate sex under the covers. Wouldn't it be great to have both? Well, you can! Even if it sounds formal at first, call your husband by his name and make him do the same to you. You will immediately notice a subtle shift in your chemistry from two cuddly, spooning mates, to two sexual beings that might actually be hot for one another.

Don't Dispense with Formalities

Megan and Brian met in their late teens and lived together for seventeen years. Megan is a music publicist and Brian a graphic artist, and they shared common interests in music and popular culture, as well as a very strong bond. They were best friends. Everyone thought they were the perfect couple, "like brother and sister" their friends used to say. In hindsight, this was *not* a good sign. Their sex life was good in the first few years, but then began to wane considerably until it only happened about once a month or less. Because the physical intimacy was so rare, Megan even considered having separate bedrooms, but she thought that might offend Brian. Even though she had turned off that side of herself, she never thought of leaving him. She and Brian were still the best of friends, and they still had so much in common. Then one day Brian woke up early in the morning crying uncontrollably. Between sobs, he said he was very sorry but he had cheated on her. Unfortunately, the girl had gotten pregnant and wanted to keep the baby even though it had been just a one-night stand. Megan was devastated and furious. And Brian was so afraid that she might actually kill him, he immediately moved in with his parents and never came back. After several months, Megan's anger had subsided and they agreed to meet at a local restaurant to chat. Although Megan knew she would never take Brian back, she still cared about him deeply and thought they could remain friends. Megan explains:

"What struck me about our first meeting after the breakup was that we actually called each other by our names. I mean, after you split up with someone, you can't keep calling him 'honey' can you? I hadn't called Brian by his real name in nearly seventeen years! When I called a girlfriend later to tell her about seeing Brian again, she thought that all I was going to talk about was his infidelity, the baby, and stuff like that. But all I could talk about was how strange it was to be calling him 'Brian' after so many years. It was like I was finally acknowledging his identity as a man again . . . like I had uncovered a part of him that had been buried for seventeen years. He hadn't called me Megan for seventeen years either. We had started calling each other 'honey' after the first couple of months we got together, then 'hun,' and then eventually 'spoon' because we loved to spoon under the covers like a couple of kids. Sometimes he was even 'papa spoon' and I was 'mama spoon.' We also talked to each other in little baby voices all the time, so it was a shock to be talking in adult tones again. I actually felt more sexual toward him that night than I had in many, many years. I realized after that meeting what a devastating toll 'honey' and those cutesy names had taken on our sex life. No wonder we hardly ever did it! I didn't excuse him for cheating on me, but I did realize that I also played a part in our sexual demise. I bet his one-night-stand girl didn't call him 'hon' or 'papa spoon!'"

Megan immediately noticed a sudden shift in the way she viewed Brian when she met with him after their breakup. Because their tone of voice was different and their cutesy names were gone, she could see him as a sexual being again. Unfortunately, in their case, it was a discovery that came too late.

Even though it may sound formal to be calling your partner by his name again, you must do it. As Megan's example shows, your relationship could depend upon it! You will gain more respect for him and he for you. Remember, you are a separate person and an adult, and because of that you shouldn't be calling each other these silly cute affectations. "Tweedle-dee" and "Tweedle-dum" are not the order of the day here. What happens when we start to call our spouse "honey" can be even more detrimental to the man than to the woman. *Honey* is not a masculine word, and that's why our husbands often become comfortable using baby voices when speaking to us at home (more on that in chapter 2).

In the beginning of any relationship, when we are still calling each other by our first names, we regard our mate as a sexual being. We are a little nervous around him, we feel very feminine around him, and we make an effort to look good in front of him. He is a man and you are a woman. Remember that first date when your eyes met and a "jolt" swept through your bodies? You felt this in all its power and sexually charged excitement. This is what life is all about, right? Now we know that it's nearly impossible to keep the giddy nervousness and excitement of the first date alive, but it *is* possible to keep the sexual tension going. And we're going to show you how to do it.

When you first started dating your husband, remember how nice it was to say his name when you spoke to him or called his work and asked for him? You probably thought, *Wow, I like this guy and I like his name, too.*

We know it's very difficult to resist the "honey brigade" around you. It's easy to call each other "honey" because everyone does it. You probably listened to your parents call each other "honey" and thought how sweet it was. All of your friends probably call their mates "honey," and they might think you're being formal if you simply call your spouse by his name. So why should you challenge the custom that the majority of couples follow? Because it will lead to more passion and sex if you do! And it will improve and deepen your relationship and the bond between you.

What's Your Sexual Dialogue?

Many women are surprised when their husbands cheat with a woman who is less attractive than they are. Why do men sometimes have sex with someone less attractive than their own wives? Because it's the mental chemistry between two people that can create sexual friction, and when that chemistry is missing at home, at least one of you is bound to find it elsewhere. Whether the third party is more attractive or less attractive than you doesn't have any bearing on sexual chemistry. For example, if another woman is calling your man by his name, looking directly into his eyes, and behaving in a confident and feminine manner, while you two are at home talking in silly voices saying "honey cakes" this and "honey pie" that, what do *you* think is going to happen? Yep, chances are that most men (and many women, too) will be tempted. By falling into the "honey" trap, the temptation to be unfaithful is greatly increased. Those of us who do cheat, more often than not, do so because the sexual dialogue between us and our partners has gone away—and it usually all started with "honey."

So, what *is* a sexual dialogue? We don't necessarily mean dirty talk in the bedroom (although sometimes that can be fun). We simply mean the way you use words, gestures, and eye contact to communicate with each other every day. This is what keeps the fires of desire burning between you—not buying sexy lingerie and planning "date nights." Dressing up in sexy lingerie or going on a date night (which most books recommend) doesn't treat the real core of sexual desire or lack of it. Sexual desire depends upon how we communicate and relate to one another, not what we happen to wear or where we happen to eat dinner. When a man or a woman strays from the relationship, it is likely because he or she is missing the sexual dialogue from the beginning of the relationship. In fact, in many cases, we don't even know what we're missing until we experience it with a stranger and then it strikes a chord within us. This experience can be very powerful and, if acted upon, can have tragic consequences—more unhappiness, extreme guilt, and possibly divorce. It may seem that looking for that missing sexual dialogue is easier with a new partner, but it really isn't.

The bottom line is this: if we don't look at why we lose our sexual dialogue, our sexual tension, and our desire for one another, we are destined to repeat the same pattern with new partners. We will live unfulfilled lives of unhappiness with one partner, or we will continually seek out new partners in a futile attempt to get that lost sexual tension back.

The following couple is a good example of two people who have completely lost their sexual dialogue with each other. Vince is an advertising executive with a large Manhattan firm, which meant he often had to entertain clients. Whenever Vince would call his wife and tell her he couldn't come home for dinner because he had to take a client out, she would say, "That's okay, honey cakes. You go ahead and keep working." And she would say this in the squeaky little-girl voice that she liked to use when talking to her husband. One night he called to tell her he had to take an important client out to the theater and then to dinner. She said, "You go ahead, honey cakes. I've got my jammies and fuzzies on [she liked to wear slippers that had fuzzy poodle faces on them], and I'll wait up for you."

When he met the client, she turned out to be a stylish brunette from London named Fiona. She called him by his formal name, Vincent, and it unexpectedly stirred something inside him. For the first time in ages, he felt like a sexual being again. His parents had named him Vincent after the legendary rocker Gene Vincent and he always preferred his formal name, even though he let his friends shorten it to Vince. During dinner, he found himself incredibly attracted to Fiona, especially the way she said his name and looked into his eyes as she spoke. He also couldn't help thinking of his wife at home "in her fuzzies" when he looked at Fiona's elegant black dress and black stiletto heels. After a few drinks she invited him to join her for coffee in her hotel suite, and they ended their evening by having passionate and out-of control sex—something he hadn't had with his wife in many years. He went home feeling incredibly guilty, of course.

His wife was waiting up for him, standing at the door, in her jammies and poodle-faced fuzzies. "Hi, honey cakes, thought you'd like some warm cocoa!" she said gleefully in her favorite little-girl voice.

What happened to Vince and his wife is very common. They had let their personas devolve into a boy-girl dynamic, instead of one appropriate to the fortysomething adults that they were. When Vince's wife called him "honey cakes," it had a subtle but very deep effect on his feelings of masculinity. His wife's little-girl persona and voice also made her seem deeply unsexual to him. How many men want to rip the clothes off a woman in "fuzzies" with a little-girl voice? Not many.

Vince later privately told us:

"Something just happened when I heard Fiona say my name several times, in that very sexy female voice of hers. It hit my brain in a different place, and I wasn't used to it. I guess it kind of awakened my 'inner male' and I felt more like a man again, instead of a little boy like I do at home."

The overriding theme in relationships like these is that once they have lost the daily sexual dialogue like Vince and his wife, it is extremely difficult to conjure up the desire for sex with their partners. By continuing to talk the way they did with one another, they had devolved into a brother/sister or boy/girl dynamic, which was definitely not sexual. Role-playing *during sex* is something that some couples may do (and this is all well and good), but Vince's wife's behavior was something very different. It wasn't creating a sexual fantasy—it had evolved out of the bedroom (where it belonged), into her daily communication and even became her everyday persona. Couples can easily fall into a familiar comfort zone with these kinds of pet names, vocal inflections and attitudes—whether it starts in the bedroom or not. Unfortunately, many don't realize the damage they are doing and probably have already done. Vince's wife may have thought her little-girl voice was cute in the bedroom and didn't see the harm in behaving this way all the time. But this seemingly innocent way of acting no longer conjured up sexual feelings from Vince for his wife. Often when one partner instigates the cutesy names and way of speaking, the other partner blindly follows . . . and the downward spiral toward a sexless marriage has begun.

During the first couple years of a relationship, *anything* can work to turn each other on because you are experiencing something (or rather some*one*) still fairly new and exciting. But the trouble starts when these habits are continued in a longer-term relationship. This is when they turn into bad habits. The reason why so many couples don't see this behavior as harmful is because anything *did* work when the relationship was still fairly new. But habits that you introduced into your relationship during the first couple of years—when you started to get a little more comfy with one another—end up doing serious damage in subsequent years. Sexual attraction can continue to be exciting in a long-term relationship, but there is a certain dynamic that needs to be adhered to when the relationship starts to pass the "newness" stage. Maybe Vince's wife's little-girl voice did turn him on at one time, but this kind of behavior doesn't stand the test of time when used in an everyday way.

Many couples have tried some of the traditional advice of other self-help books but sadly, it didn't change a thing in their sex lives. This is because the advice offered didn't get to the real problem in the first place—a couple's daily bad habits with one another. By continuing these bad habits from earlier in the relationship, they unknowingly damage their sexual chemistry even further. In fact, the advice from these other books is like taking your car to a mechanic because the engine isn't running well, only to have him tell you, "Give it a new coat of paint and it will run great!" This next couple tried the advice that so many self-help sex books recommend—concentrating on the paint job rather than looking under the hood.

The Not-So-Sexy Sex Weekend

"My husband and I have a great marriage . . . I think," said Irma, an attractive woman in her thirties who's been happily married to her husband, Guy, for eight years. She continues:

"We love our son, Dashiel, so much. He's three years old and a handful, of course, but the joy and fun he has brought to our lives is immeasurable. When Dash was born, our sex life went dormant in the first year, which is like most couples, I suppose. We were so overwhelmed with all of the work and the emotions that come with bringing a new life into the world, we didn't get back on a sexual footing at all. Not that we didn't think about it. We'd joke about the fact that our sex life was 'in the toilet' but we really didn't worry about it either because everything else in the marriage was going so great—our new son was amazing, our first home was beautiful, and both our jobs were going great, too. With everything going so well, I thought, *Why should I complain about sex? It will take care of itself.* But it didn't. So I ended up buying lots of self-help books to see what we could do. Guy was great about it, and so we started to try different things.

"One Friday afternoon we dropped Dashiel off at his Grandma's so we could have a 'sex weekend.' I bought lots of new lingerie, and we even bought new satin sheets. The weekend went okay. We did have intercourse once, but I unfortunately couldn't reach an orgasm—I think because it was so long since I'd even masturbated that I had forgotten how to do it. So although it was a fun two days, I certainly wouldn't call it a 'sex weekend.' We spent most of the time watching old movies and eating pizza in bed, which was great, but we ended up just doing a lot of spooning and hugging. I mean, compared to most couples I know, I feel like I should be grateful that we can spend a really fun weekend together in bed. A lot of my friends couldn't even do that without getting bored or getting into a fight about something. So right now we're just happy to be cuddling a lot. Maybe sometime in the future the hot sex we had in the beginning will come back . . . that's what I'm hoping for anyway."

We asked Irma what she and her husband call each other at home and out in public. She said:

"Well, in public we call each other 'honey' but at home he's 'poopie' and I'm 'moopie'—kind of our version of mommy and daddy, I guess. When we had our sex weekend together, Guy would say something like, 'Does moopie want that special kind of cuddle?' Guess it's not super sensual is it?"

No, it isn't. Most couples don't realize the destructive power of these cute pet names. They don't even realize that it's happening at all. Like Irma and Guy, they are usually very puzzled as to why they don't feel sexual, but they resign themselves to thinking this is normal in a relationship.

Sadly, most couples feel powerless to change a sexless period in their lives, and they simply wait for it to pass, which rarely happens. The fact is, every time we use those pet names, day in and day out, we weaken our sexual selves. Imagine a horse and cart traveling down the same muddy road day after day. Eventually the tracks get so deep that the cart is literally stuck in a rut and can't easily change direction. Similarly, how are you then going to switch your brain into sex mode when it's been in "honey" mode day after day?

The Ol' Ball and Chain

Sometimes those supposedly sweet terms of endearment can take a turn for the worse and be not so endearing. And this is even more destructive. Some couples can call each other names that are downright rude, crude, and even abusive. Even if the offended partner accepts this behavior, it's usually because the other partner says it's "all in fun." For instance, how many of us have heard someone call his wife "the ol' ball and chain?" Words have a deep impact on our psyche, and the constant repetition of names like these does not encourage a loving and sexual relationship, or a good sense of self-esteem.

In Spanish, for instance, it's very common for spouses to call each other *gorda* or *gordo*, which means "fat one." We spoke to several people who said that their parents would use these terms of "affection" with them when they were children too, often calling them *gordito* or *gordita* (little fat one). One woman even told us that she eventually became anorexic because she grew up feeling like she was always going to be a *gordita*. She never felt she could be thin enough, even when she weighed less than a hundred pounds. Even the words *feo* (ugly) and *enano* (short person) are sometimes used as terms of endearment in Spanish, both for children and for spouses. But what does this do to someone when they hear themselves called this day after day? And what kind of image does it leave in the mind of the person using the term? If your partner is going to call you "my little fatty" day in and day out, don't you think that in his mind, you eventually *become* a "little fatty"? It affects both people in the relationship. Even though some people will say they're "used to it," or it doesn't bother them too much, is it really a practice that should be accepted? We don't think so.

If you met someone on a blind date and he started calling you "gorda," wouldn't you want to slap him across the face? So why do we let words like this be used every day just because we happen to know someone well? It's simply not acceptable. Similarly, if you start dating a guy and he introduces you to his friends as his "old lady" or his "ball and chain" wouldn't you be offended? Hell yeah! Hearing yourself called "old lady" day after day is not going to make you feel sexy, vibrant, and young, is it? And I'm sure that your mate doesn't really like being referred to as an "old man" either. Words are important. They can carry a lot of weight, especially when repeated. They settle in parts of our brain and can have a huge impact on how we view ourselves and how we view our relationship with our partner. And often, the more we hear ourselves called a certain word, the more we come to believe that it must be true— just like the one hundred–pound "gordita."

We spoke to one woman in her fifties named Olivia, a mother of three beautiful teenage daughters, who probably had to endure the worst so-called term of endearment that we'd ever heard before.

"After I went through menopause a couple of years ago, my husband, Doug, started calling me his 'dead vessel' around the house. Even my daughters thought it was funny at first, so I went along with his little joke. Eventually though, it really started to bother me. I mean, menopause was actually a very painful time for me emotionally. I really did feel like an important part of me as a woman was dead. So I finally ended up telling Doug to stop. And do you know what he said to me? He said I just didn't have a sense of humor! He still calls me 'dead vessel' every once in a while, even though he knows it still bothers me. He especially makes a point to do it when one of the kids is around because he thinks it'll get a laugh out of them. I really hate it. I don't get the humor in it at all, and it makes me so angry and totally resentful that he still does it. Even if it's just once in a while, it still really hurts my feelings. Normally we have a pretty good partnership and he's been such a great dad with the girls, but his so-called sense of humor really isn't that funny. Whenever he calls me that stupid nick-name, I'm tempted to start calling him something like 'princess tiny meat,' or 'needle dick,' or 'Mr. Softie,' or even the totally apathetic term 'sperm donor!' I wonder how he'd feel if I started calling him stuff like that, now and then?!"

We didn't ask Olivia how her sex life was these days. Frankly, we already knew the answer. Being called a "dead vessel" clearly didn't make her feel like a sexy woman. She seemed to have so much built-up resentment against Doug that we sincerely doubt there's much sex going on in that household. Sex and resentment are never a great combo.

From Primal to Preschool

Nicknames for each other are not good for your relationship, whether they sound cruel or cute. It may have been "lotsa" fun in preschool, but not now, when you are both supposed to be two sexual adults, as the following couple illustrates.

Ted and Mindy, who have been living together for over ten years, are another couple for whom using the word *honey* has led to sexual problems. Neither of them ever wanted to have children, and so they have a lot of free time to pursue their shared interests. They have four dogs—all rescued from a local shelter—and they spend much of their free time taking the dogs on hiking trips and to the local dog parks. They both love the outdoors and spend at least one weekend a month in their motor home, traveling to new locations in the desert or the mountains, along with their beloved dogs. Even though their sex life is not what it used to be, they are still best friends and neither of them has ever thought of cheating. Mindy recalls:

"In the beginning, Ted was the most masculine guy I had ever met. He was my ideal man. He works in construction and used to play college football, so his body has always been very muscular and toned. When I first met him, I thought *Wow! He's the perfect guy for me.* A macho Michael Madsen type, but very sweet and shy. I'll never forget one of the first times we made love. While we were taking a shower together, Ted looked into my eyes without smiling. The look was, 'I'm going to fuck you, and I can't wait to do it.' It was the sexiest look any man had ever given me! His eyes were boring into me—like a wild animal, he had captured me and wasn't going to let me go. He was so masculine, so dominant, and so primal. He just kept looking into my eyes without smiling, but gently rubbing my back, my breasts, then my pussy. Then he said, 'God, Mindy, you are so sexy.' The way he said my name just then, all low and guttural, I practically had an orgasm in the shower before we even started having sex! It was the most erotic moment in my entire life.

"We continued to have a really hot sex life in the first couple of years, but then for some reason, we started to become more best friends than lovers. We began to call each other 'honey,' like most couples, and then soon after, Ted started to call sex 'coochie.' I thought it was kind of cute at first, and then it just stuck. If he wanted to have sex, Ted would say, 'Does honey want *coochie* tonight?' Even I started using the word. But looking back on it, when we started to call each other 'honey' and use the word coochie for sex, we ended up having less and less of it.

"I still can't believe that this is the same guy who gave me that look in the shower years ago and said my name the way he did. That guy wanted to 'take me' big time, but the guy I have now wants to have 'coochie with his honey.' Somehow he's lost that super-primal masculinity that he had in the beginning, and I'm not sure how he can get it back. In fact, because I see him as my all-too-familiar 'honey,' I just can't seem to get excited enough to want to have sex with him very much. Now he's just my 'honey,' you know?"

When your partner starts to use cutesy words for sex, tell him that you would prefer him to say he wants to "make love to you," "have sex with you," or simply "fuck you." Do not do the Ted and Mindy thing and use cutesy words for each other or for sex. Sex is sexy. Sex is hot. Sex is *not* "coochie!" Their relationship was so hot and so healthy in the beginning, but sadly, they sabotaged it by using words like *honey* and *coochie*.

So let's start by thinking how you would act if you had met your mate for the first time. Put yourself in that place again and act on it. In the beginning you called each other by your first names, right? And you didn't use those cutesy words for sex either. For instance, would your new lover say in bed, "Honey, do you feel like coochie tonight?" We think not. Calling each other by your proper names is the first place to start. It may sound like an insignificant step, but believe us, it's not. Names and words have a very deep and lasting impact, so trust in the process. It may feel strange at first, like you are backtracking in your relationship, but it *will* work! Sometimes you have to go backwards to move forward in the right way.

So, don't be afraid to start calling each other by your names. You need to be vigilant, though, and never let another "honey" be spoken in your household, unless you're speaking to your dog. Banish the word *honey* forever. Correct your partner if he starts to call you *any* term of endearment. Habits that you've built up over the years are very hard to break, we know. But it will be worth it. Soon you'll notice the subtle difference in your sexual chemistry. Your husband won't seem like just a "cuddly, teddy bear, spoon-mate" to you, but the masculine lover that he once was and still can be. He will per-ceive you differently too. Not as the "honey" waiting at home in your "fuzzies," but as the sensual, female lover that you know inside you still are.

Give yourselves time to allow your sexual subconscious to respond to calling each other by your proper names. The power of words is truly amazing. From the destructive nature of calling each other "honey" to the restorative nature of calling each other your individual names, you need to give your mind the time to let those changes happen. You can't force sexual attraction and desire. But if you change the way you address one another, your brain will do the rest—without you even realizing it. Yes, it's easy to call each other "honey" because everyone does it. But if you take the road less traveled and stop calling him "honey" you will be profoundly and pleasurably rewarded. We promise.

STAYING OUT OF THE HONEY TRAP

1 Stop calling him sweet, androgynous names like "honey," "sweetie," and "pookie." And yes, even the ultra-cute "schmoopy" must be banished!

2 Remember that there is sexual potency in using your proper names. Male and female. Man and woman. Relish the power, importance, and sexuality of your names.

3 Don't allow sex to have a cutesy name either. "Coochie," for example, is not sexy and will not make you hot for one another.

4 Take your thoughts of your partner back to the beginning, before you got too comfy with each other and introduced those bad habits. Start from there and enjoy the newness again.

5 Allow the power of calling each other by your names again to wash over you and open the floodgates to your new sexual dialogue.

Chapter Two

Banish the Baby Talk

"There's nothing more unsexy than hearing a man talk in a squeaky, baby voice, having a conversation with his wife."

—SAMANTHA, AGE 42

"Ever since we had our baby, my husband calls me Mommy. And I know it shouldn't bother me, but it kinda does."

—HEIDI, AGE 32

IN THE PREVIOUS CHAPTER, we showed that calling each other "honey" usually degenerates into more childish names like "papa and mama spoon," and the truly pathetic "moopie and poopie." And along with these cutesy names usually comes a squeaky change in voice pitch, from that of a normal adult to something akin to a three-year-old child's . . . the dreaded "baby talk." Why does this happen? Well, it's because once Pandora's box is opened with "honey," bad habits will arrive that can become even more entrenched in our daily lives. We've all heard baby talk between couples we know or have even done it ourselves. Sadly, this is another way of causing a detrimental shift in the relationship. It can change us from sexual adults to asexual young juveniles, or even worse, it can create a mother/son or father/daughter dynamic between a couple. Using baby talk is another deadly killer of sexual desire.

Baby talk happens with couples young and old, rich or poor. Even the most powerful people in the world have done it. For instance, even former President Reagan would often refer to his wife Nancy as "Mommy" (*The Reagan Diaries* by Ronald Reagan). And this was one of the most powerful men in the world at the time calling his wife "Mommy"! You see how common this stuff is?

If this kind of talk is in your relationship, you need to change the habit immediately. It's not harmless, it's not cute, and it's certainly not sexy. Baby talk is another way that couples inadvertently desexualize their relationship without even realizing that it's happening, as the following story illustrates.

Me and Mrs. Jones . . .

Janet and Casey had been living together for twelve years. Janet told us that in the first few years, their sex life was great. She would plan sex nights several days in advance and the anticipation would make the night more exciting when it finally arrived. Then they had their first child, a beautiful son named Adam, and everything changed. The sex-night ritual went out the door. Janet is a teacher, and Casey is a bank manager—both very demanding full-time jobs. With the overwhelming responsibilities of a new baby, they didn't feel they had enough time or energy to devote to their sex life. To make matters worse, Janet started calling Casey "Daddy" and Casey started calling Janet "Mommy." They just couldn't help it, they said. Since Janet used baby talk with their newborn son, she started using the same squeaky, baby voice at home all of the time, even when speaking with Casey. They both saw it as playful and cute, and didn't think anything of it.

Until Janet began to wonder, when was the last time they had sex? By the time Adam was three years old, Janet told us that she calculated that they hadn't had sex more than a handful of times since his birth. Her girlfriends told her she shouldn't worry about it, though. They told her that it's normal to stop having sex when a baby comes along, especially when it's a couple's firstborn. However normal some people think it is, though, this kind of sexual drought doesn't just take care of itself. The cause of this common dilemma wasn't just the new child in their lives, but it was also a result of how Janet and Casey's communication with each other changed after they became parents.

One afternoon, while Janet was picking up Adam from the day care center, she started chatting with a single dad about his daughter, who liked to play with her son. She was intrigued by his deep, sexy voice and the way he said her name. She admitted to us that it was at that moment that she felt a jolt of sexual attraction.

"He used to be a radio disc jockey, and I know it sounds corny, but his voice was like velvet to my ears. Each time I would drop Adam off at day care, I started looking for this guy. Even now, I don't want to say his name because I still feel so guilty about it. Sometimes I even waited in my car up to an hour, just so I could run into him. I started to feel like I was stalking him, but I just couldn't stop! Though it was sometimes as much as ninety degrees outside, I waited in my car with the engine running and the air conditioner on, just so I could see him and talk to him when he arrived. I felt I had to see him, or I would be depressed for the rest of the day. Each time we met and spoke for a few minutes, I noticed that we started to talk more about our personal lives and less about our kids.

"I was becoming so obsessed with him that seeing him for those few moments at day care wasn't enough anymore. So one morning I asked him out for coffee—knowing full well I was going further in the direction of possibly cheating on Casey. I felt guilty and scared, worried that we might run into someone we knew. He told me he lived alone, was recently divorced, and that he took care of his daughter nine months out of the year. He definitely let me know he wasn't seeing anyone. As the weeks rolled on, I met him several times at the same local coffee bar, and each time I found myself becoming more and more attracted to him. He knew I was married, of course, but he wanted to keep seeing me anyway, even if it was only for coffee. I must say, I felt like a woman again, just by the way he talked to me and stared into my eyes.

"I realized that I was heading towards infidelity when I found myself masturbating in the mornings after Casey got out of bed, all the while thinking of this man from the day care center. But I couldn't understand why I was doing this! Why was I contemplating risking my relationship and family for a man I barely knew? Looking back on it now, I realize that he wasn't any more handsome than Casey. He wasn't as funny as Casey either. He wasn't even as interesting as Casey. But there was just something about the way he made me feel that hooked me beyond my control.

"One day when we were at the coffee bar, he kissed me and started stroking my back. I was so turned on—we both were—that we starting planning how we could spend some alone time together during the day. Somewhere private. Just then, out of the corner of my eye, I saw the wife of Casey's best friend staring at us from across the coffee bar. She quickly looked away and left. She didn't say hello or come over—and this was a woman who had been to my house many times—so who knows how long she had been watching us or what she was thinking! One thing I knew for certain, though, was that her husband was definitely going to find out about us, probably as soon as she got to her car and used her cell phone.

"I panicked and quickly left as well. When I saw Casey at the end of the day, I knew I had to confess to him. I was so afraid when he came home because I thought he might already know everything. His friend was bound to tell him that his wife saw me looking very intimate with another man. And even if he didn't say anything to Casey, I didn't like the idea that couples we knew might gossip about me behind his back. I didn't want to put him in that situation. I really respect and love Casey. So that night I told him everything—how I had met this man several times, how I was attracted to him, and even how we were planning to meet at a motel soon. Casey was pretty devastated. I never want to see that look of hurt on his face ever again, believe me. He went to bed sobbing, and it wasn't until a few days later that we started to talk about it.

"When we did finally talk about it, amazingly, one of the first things Casey said was 'Well, I guess something like this was bound to happen, since neither of us have been acting like lovers for a long time. I'm just glad Dan's wife saw you that day. I think she was meant to be there—because if you had taken it further, I think our relationship would have been over.' Casey was so great. He forgave me, but not without a lot of pain and tears. I get teary-eyed now just thinking of it. We talked a lot about our sex life and how it had gotten away from us, and we both said we wanted to make a real effort to get ourselves in a sexual place again. The first thing we did was go away for a weekend, without Adam, and we had the most emotional and loving sex that we'd ever had in our twelve years together. It was really beautiful.

"It's weird, because when all of this happened, Casey and I stopped calling each other 'Mommy' and 'Daddy,' and speaking in baby voices to each other. I suppose you can't really do that after you've been through such a painful experience. I felt a change right away in how I felt about Casey, just because we weren't using baby talk anymore. It was like our sexual selves were given a chance to breathe again. After a couple of weeks of talking like adults, I told Casey that I never wanted go back to the stupid 'Mommy/Daddy' stuff, and he agreed. Looking back on it, I think the main thing that attracted me to the day care guy was just the experience of relating to a man as a woman again. I've run into him several times since and to tell you the truth, I really don't know what I ever saw in him. I think I was just longing to have a man speak to me like an adult."

Only after Janet stopped using baby talk with Casey did she realize what a toll it had taken on their sex lives, and how close she had come to needlessly throwing away their relationship as a result. As with the story in the previous chapter of Vince and his wife in her "fuzzies," Janet didn't realize what was missing in her relationship with Casey until she experienced it with a stranger. And because of chance circumstances, she was thankfully able to stop this relationship with the other man before it went any further. What many couples don't realize is that the tone and words in which they speak to one another has a *huge* impact on their sexual chemistry. For Janet and Casey, having a child inadvertently caused them to change their way of speaking from lovers and life partners, to "Mommy" and "Daddy." This can seem harmless at the time, and if anything, may even seem like the logical step for new parents. Like any relationship, their way of relating to each other is constantly evolving. And, of course, their new and wonderful relationship with their child does have a big impact on that. We know that priorities change when a child comes into the picture. You have become "mommies" and "daddies." But it is important to always remember—you are a "mommy" and a "daddy" to your children, not to each other.

Even in relationships where there are no children, couples can still fall into this bad habit. And oftentimes it can be the husband and not the wife who is guilty of this practice. We have found that husbands tend to be more prone to use baby talk than their wives. Many men seem to be still looking for a mother figure in their lives, even though they are now adults. When they get married, they can sometimes transfer the same kind of affection they had toward their mother to their new wife. It is understandable that this could easily happen, as the role of the woman in a long-term relationship tends to include things like cooking, doing the laundry and ironing, cleaning the house, and generally caring for the man. Of course, it would be wonderful if every man wanted to share in these chores or even do them entirely—we can all dream, right? But that is not the traditional dynamic. It may even be that you tried to get him to do stuff around the house, like the dishes or vacuuming. But maybe he's not as thorough as you, and you like it done "just so." (We both wonder if sometimes men purposely do these chores badly, so that we women end up doing it anyway!) At the end of the day, in all relationships, there are various roles that evolve in the daily goings-on that might give the impression of caregiver, or someone's "mommy" or "'daddy." But regardless of who does what in your household, here's the important thing to note: these are simply chores to make your daily lives run smoothly. That's all. They are not invitations to view one another differently than the lovers you started out to be and hopefully still are.

In many countries, men often go directly from living in their parents' home—with their mother doing their laundry and taking care of them—to getting married and living with their wife, who also ends up taking care of them. What can happen in these situations is that the wife becomes the new mother figure for the man. After all, she takes care of him, washes his clothes, cleans the house, prepares his meals—all the things his mother used to do. Except, husbands and wives have sex . . . at least that is what is supposed to happen, right? But, when a baby comes along, or even before a baby comes along, the new husband may look for a girlfriend. Not that he wants to leave his wife—he doesn't. His wife is now the center of his life and the center of his family. But, unfortunately, she is not the center of his sexuality anymore. The wife now does the motherly duties around the house, and in her husband's mind, she has become "Mommy."

This kind of dynamic may confirm to him, and to you, that your relationship is no longer sexual. You have now become his surrogate mother and caregiver. Hence, the former "husband" and now "son" will search for a girlfriend. And ironically, the girlfriend may even be married herself! But because she is not cooking his meals, doing his laundry, and generally caring for his daily practical needs, he sees her as a sexual being and not as a mother figure. Simply put, men have very deep emotions and perceptions regarding the role of wife and mother, whether conscious or not, and these feelings can often play havoc with a couple's sex life.

The Oedipus Complex

Oedipus was a mythical Greek character who killed his father and married his mother—albeit unknowingly. (Really, not a super-sweet guy!) Over the years, many professionals in the psychiatric field have made many inferences and conclusions from this fable. Sigmund Freud once wrote about it this way: "It is the fate of all of us, perhaps, to direct our first sexual impulse towards our mother and our first hatred and our first murderous wish against our father."

We don't want to get all Freudian here, but the important thing to gain from Freud's theories and the so-called Oedipus Complex is that a man's relationship with his mother is indeed very complex. When you become a mother yourself (or even when you are only acting in a motherly role around the house) this often triggers behaviors and feelings in your partner that are rooted in his childhood. Some men even have a hard time thinking of their wives as sexual beings after they have given birth. Your new motherhood can remind him of feelings he had for his own mother, and most men don't think of their mothers in sexual terms, as least not consciously. Your husband might respect you and even idolize you once he has seen you perform the miracle of childbirth, but sometimes these new feelings can also kill the sexual sparks in his head.

Of course we acknowledge that not only can it be difficult for your husband to think of you as a sexual creature again after giving birth, it can also be extremely hard for you to feel sexual as well. You're tired, your breasts ache, your body doesn't feel or look the same—and you've got this amazing new life form that needs you and is constantly demanding of your attention. Having a child is one of the most fulfilling experiences in life. Unfortunately, though, it is also so emotionally and physically overwhelming that we sometimes lose sight of ourselves in the process.

However, as modern women, we should not allow this to happen. This may sound harsh to say, but your life is not your child. Sure, you would give your life up for your child if he or she was in physical danger. But this doesn't mean, in normal circumstances, that you should give the entirety of your life up for your child. How many of us let our children sleep in our bed, long after it's normal to do so? How many of us neglect our husbands, neglect our friends, and most important, neglect ourselves when a child comes into our lives? It's very, very common.

Gimme a Break, Why Don't Cha?

Nina is a new mother in her early thirties and she explained to us one night how motherhood changed her life in ways she didn't anticipate:

"When Joshua was born two years ago, everything changed—how I felt about my body, how I felt about sex, and also how I felt about my husband Joe. I think Joe and I had a good sex life up until then. We'd been together eight years and still loved sex, but when Joshua came along, sex was the *last* thing on my mind. Also, I felt like Joe's life went along pretty much the same as before: he still worked the same hours, he still played golf once a week, he even still went to happy hour with his work buddies on Fridays. But my life totally changed, and I probably felt some resentment about that. My body changed, my schedule changed, and the emotional and physical attachment to Joshua was much more powerful than I had ever expected. I didn't care about Joe anymore, I didn't care about my friends—all I could think about was Joshua. Joe started to feel neglected, physically and emotionally. He also started to use a baby voice around the house, and he started to call me 'Mommy,' which totally creeped me out. I told him to stop all of that, and thankfully he did, but he still acted like a whiny child sometimes, someone who needed me for comfort. But no one was there to comfort me. I felt like I had two babies, instead of one!"

Women are not only the physical life force in the world, but they are usually the emotional heart and soul of the family. One mother we spoke with said that she could never reveal that she was a little depressed (however infrequent) in front of her teenage daughters or her husband. She said that her family seemed to depend upon her always being her usual "bubbly" self for them to feel content. And whenever she wasn't feeling that great, she had to pretend otherwise or they would "freak out." That position in the center of the family can often be extremely draining for a woman. It can also leave her little time for herself, as Nina soon came to realize:

"After a couple of years of hardly any sex and me never leaving the house because I didn't trust the babysitters, I began to feel really depressed. I knew I had to make some changes. I realized I was letting motherhood swallow up my whole life, something I knew my mother did as well. She never had any friends or hobbies, and she never showed any affection for my father either. Although I know she loved us, she showed it in a way that was kind of smothering—something I really noticed when I was a teenager. She wanted to be my best friend, and I think she got jealous when I had my own school friends and didn't always want her with me. I remember she also got really sad when my brother had a steady girlfriend in high school. And God, you should have seen her the day my brother got married! Her face was so long, she looked like she was at a funeral, not a wedding! I think her life totally revolved around us, which wasn't good for her at all. And when my brother and I got older, it wasn't good for us either.

"So I said to Joe, 'I'm getting a babysitter and we're going on a spa vacation!' 'Cool!' he said. We went to this luxurious spa in the desert outside of Los Angeles, and even though it was summertime, we loved it. The extreme heat made the whole vacation seem even sexier. Joe was great. He never even approached me for sex because I think he knew I just really needed to rest. He didn't act like the whiny child that he sometimes did at home either. I had a facial, two massages, and we spent time at night in the hot mineral pool, just lying back and holding hands. I think because Joe really just catered to me for a change and wasn't thinking about his own needs, it made me want him again, more than I had in at least two years. We made love several times during that trip, and it was really hot—both temperature-wise and sexually! I think because I stood up and said I needed to take care of myself, it made him want to take care of me, instead of me always being the caregiver. His whiny child went back in the closet, thank God. I wish he would have suggested the spa vacation himself, but I think sometimes men don't even realize how overworked we are as mothers.

"Now that I have expressed my need to be taken care of, Joe knows that I need a break from motherhood every now and then. When I'm not happy with how I'm feeling, I'm going to stand up and make sure my needs are met. For Joe, for Joshua, and for myself. Now we get a babysitter at least once a week, and I really feel like I'm getting my life back again. I've started to do volunteer work for the local animal shelter on Sunday afternoons, which has really been great for me because I love animals. Joshua is still everything to me, of course. Even more so now. I love him dearly. But I realize now that loving him doesn't have to mean I forget about myself.

"I think my mother was a great mother, but I think she was

kind of a martyr, too. She always let my brother and I know that she gave up a lot to raise us. I remember she always used to remind us that she never finished art college because we came along. I never want Joshua to think I gave up my life for him. He's an amazing addition to my life. But he's not my whole life."

It's hard to reward and pamper yourself when you think your total self-worth is your role as mother and/or homemaker. In the case of Nina and Joe, she clearly needed to give herself a break and enjoy her life a bit more. She was at a physical and emotional breaking point before she even gave herself some slack and asked for help. Even if your husband works and you are a homemaker, you still need to stand up for yourself and say as Nina did, "I need a vacation, and I need a babysitter!" Continue to find ways to get out of that "mother only" mind-set. If that means bringing in a cleaning service now and then, or getting your husband to help you with housework some-times, then do it. This is a necessary thing to ensure that the two of you remain the adult sexual partners that you should be.

Mario and His Mamacita

Diane is a forty-year-old new mom in San Diego. She met her husband, Mario, ten years ago when they both were in the military. They lived in a very spacious new home in a beautiful coastal com-munity with their one-year-old daughter, Lily. Diane was happy to give up her career once she became pregnant because she had always wanted to be a full-time mother. She had grown up in a foster home in Texas and never knew her own parents, so she was determined to give her daughter a much different upbringing than the one she had experienced.

"Mario and I always had a very close relationship, especially since we both had careers in the military. Even though Mario hadn't grown up in a foster home as I had, I knew he didn't have a perfect childhood. He grew up in a house with seven children and no father. His mother, his grandmother, and his aunt kept the family together with a lot of love but not always much money. We both came up the hard way, and I think that made us even closer. He adored his mother, and I did too. She was so sweet and so hardworking. I remember Mario telling me that at one time, his mother worked three jobs to save enough for the down payment on a house. He said that his mother worked so hard that sometimes she would only come home to have breakfast with them before going off to work. When she slept, he never knew.

"When Mario and I got married and moved in together five years ago, I noticed that things started changing in the relationship. He was expecting me to do his laundry and cook his meals, in a very sweet but also very persuasive way. When I finally got pregnant two years ago, things really changed. He started calling me 'Momacita' instead of 'honey' or the usual pet names we had for each other. I used to tell him, 'Hey, I don't even speak Spanish, so I don't think I'm your 'Mamacita!' But he wouldn't stop, and 'Momacita' became my new name, and he adopted this squeaky babylike voice that he started to use around the house. Our daughter was born a little over a year ago, and we haven't made love since she was born. I

found out a few months ago from a friend who still works in the military that he has had a girlfriend for the last two years—ever since he started calling me 'Mamacita.'
I really think that once I became a mother, he just didn't see me as sexual partner anymore. I just couldn't handle that he was being unfaithful, especially since we just had a baby. So we separated.

"I just saw Mario last week when he came to pick up Lily, and he told me that his relationship with his girlfriend is now over, and he wants to come back to me. He's currently living on the base, and we're going through counseling together, which has been really draining. I hope we can work things out and live together again. I do miss him and I know Lily does too. But a lot of stuff has come up in therapy regarding his feelings about motherhood and sexuality, which has been a real eye-opener, believe me. I told him in therapy that I really think the baby voices and the 'Mamacita' stuff didn't help our sex life or our relationship, and I think he's finally starting to understand."

When Mario began using the squeaky-voiced baby talk, he was confirming to himself and to Diane that she was now his "Mamacita" and not his sexual partner anymore. We all need to be aware of this when it starts to occur. As women, we need to guard our position in the marriage as our husband's sexual and *equal* partner. Don't allow your husband to unwittingly "baby talk" the sexual relationship away. In the case of Mario and Diane, Mario may not have even wanted to have a girlfriend, but because he had programmed himself to consider his wife as "Momacita," he began to feel unfulfilled as a sexual man. This then facilitated his need to look for a sexual partner somewhere else. Diane did all she could to get him to quit this behavior, but unlike Nina's husband, he just wouldn't stop.

Men can be very persuasive, and can sometimes alter our perception of ourselves as women and the kind of role we play in the household. Many of us have grown up in families where our mothers had to compromise in a big or even a small way, and it's still difficult for us as women to not compromise at all. But you need to remember that there are certain things in the relationship that are nonnegotiable. You are not his mother, you are not his housekeeper, you are not his caregiver, and you are not his sibling. Even if you have to fight about it, so be it! You are his sexual partner and his life partner, period!

Papa's Got a Brand New Bag

Not all relationships are traditional in this way, however. Quite often in our modern society, there are some role reversals, and with that can come some similar issues. John, forty-two, and Cynthia, forty, are a good example of a couple who has a nontraditional home life. Yet the roles they took in the household affected their sexual roles, much the same way if they had been a more traditional couple. They have been together for fifteen years and until fairly recently, they both had full-time, very fulfilling careers—John, as an architect, and Cynthia as an advertising executive. For most of that time they had a fairly healthy sex life—until about five years ago, when they decided to try to have a child. Unfortunately, after many attempts, they found they weren't able to have a child by natural means and resorted to IVF treatments. The stress of trying so hard to get pregnant took its toll on the fun aspect of their sex life, Cynthia told us. But they discussed and accepted this, and figured that it would get better again once they had gone through this difficult and stressful hurdle. They were finally blessed with not one but two children: beautiful twin girls. Because Cynthia's career was the much higher-paying one, it was decided between them that John would put his career on hold and stay home with the girls during their formative years. They figured that once they settled into a good routine, they could try to put some fun back into their sex life. Cynthia explains:

"We discussed it extensively, and reached a decision that because my job was more steady and higher paying, John would stay home with the kids. What I found was that although I looked up to John before and saw him as an intelligent man—my man—I now started looking at him and treating him differently once he became a stay-at-home dad. I don't know why I did this, but I started calling him 'Mommy' as a little joke and sometimes kind of belittling him. For some reason I would really talk down to him. I couldn't understand why I was treating him differently just because he was staying at home, but I guess it was a subconscious thing considering how I was brought up, which was in a very traditional family. You know, the typical family, with Mom staying at home with us kids and Dad working full time and 'bringing home the bacon.' So, even though this decision for John to be the one to stay at home was mutual and I fully agreed with it, it started playing with my head. We really didn't have sex much at all after the kids were born. And, if I'm to be honest with myself, I was seeing him as an emasculated man and because of that I was losing respect for him. And because of that lack of respect, he wasn't turning me on anymore. We started fighting more too. I feel myself drifting away from him, but I just don't know how to remedy it."

In the case of John and Cynthia, they found themselves in a situation that was unavoidable for financial reasons. There are a lot of modern couples also finding themselves in this same position. Some couples aren't affected by the role reversal, but some are. In the same way as Mario should have done, Cynthia needs to make a concerted effort to not talk to John in a "babying" way. For Cynthia, calling John "Mommy" is quite damaging to his male ego. John needs to take his power back as a man and to insist that they use adult voices and their real names with each other again. And sexually, John needs to take on the role as the traditional man again. He needs to show that in the area of their personal relationship together, he *is* still the man. You must never lose sight of your identity as a man or a woman, regardless of the roles taken in bringing up your kids. Those identities need to be established and respected.

Now, although it can be common for men to resort to those little squeaky voices, women are not exempt from this bad behavior at all! Hence, the following scenario about Lucy and Dalton. Both in their midtwenties, Lucy and Dalton were together four years and married for two of those years. Lucy, a fashion buyer for a department store, and Dalton, a contractor, had a pretty normal, healthy sex life when they were first together. But like so many long-term relationships, things started to change.

"For the first one and a half years we were going out, Dalton and I really loved each other and we had a great relationship. That's why we decided to take it to the next step and get married. Unfortunately though, once we moved in together, we started treating each other differently. I have to admit now that I kinda allowed it to happen as much as Dalton did. You see, I'm from a pretty traditional, strict family, and so is he. We were both still living with our parents the whole time we were dating and even after we were engaged. Because we knew that our parents wouldn't be happy about us sleeping together in their house, we had to get creative about finding places to be alone together back then. Dalton had an SUV, and we'd park on a small dark street some nights and just do it frantically in the back. It was fun and exciting and definitely hot! But, I guess when we got married, all our preconceptions of how a wife and husband should behave came out without us really even realizing it. Of course, it came from what we saw growing up. My mother was pretty meek in her relationship and was a stay-at-home mom, while my Dad was pretty controlling and a little overbearing. And Dalton's family life was exactly the same, which was probably one of the reasons we thought we were so perfectly matched.

"The difference was that although we had a similar family upbringing, I had actually done more in my life and career than both our mothers in many respects. I graduated college with a degree in fashion merchandising, and with the exception of still living at home, I was actually a pretty independent woman. But somehow it all changed when we got married.

Dalton would insist on doing everything important—'now that I'm the husband,' he would say. So he'd do all the bills, everything to do with the now joint bank account, and basically everything else that wasn't cooking or cleaning. And I even had a weekly allowance. He would tell me, 'Oh you can just run around the house barefoot and be the "little wifey," and I'll take care of everything, "puss-puss."' So I just became 'the little wifey' and let him take over. And then, for some strange reason, I started to become this 'wittle helpless girl' that couldn't do anything without her 'dawg-dawg.' It got to the point where whenever we would have sex, I'd start talking like this little five-year-old girl, all helpless and all like, 'Ooh, does big dawgie want me to get on my knees and suck on his big Popsicle?' The bedroom role-playing got so commonplace that we ended up acting that way all the time.

"Looking back now, I'm pretty disgusted at my behavior really. Because it was kinda sick, huh? I mean, it was almost bordering on pedophilia! Before we got married, I was his equal—his sexual equal and his female counterpart. But from then on, it just continued to go even more downhill. The more I spoke in my helpless little-girl voice, the more controlling and 'daddylike' he became. After a year of that, we stopped having sex altogether, because frankly, I think I started hating myself and I also resented feeling like I was this kept woman—or should I say child! I had lost respect for myself and he definitely had too. I think at first he liked his 'wittle girl', but after a while his little girl became more of a sullen, whiny child that he didn't want to be around. The worst thing was, we both had become so used to treating each other like 'big daddy' and 'helpless little girl,' we didn't know how to get out of it. We split up just a few months ago, and there's just so much crap under the bridge now, we can't even talk to one another anymore. It's amazing to me what our stupid preconceptions of husband and wife turned us into. If only we had known what that kind of baby talk and father/daughter stuff could do to our relationship, maybe we could have saved it."

What happened to Lucy and Dalton was such a shame, as they had a good relationship to begin with. Though Lucy's little-girl persona was indeed pretty extreme, many of us are guilty of the same thing, but just to a lesser degree. Even though it may have been common for women years ago to use a little-girl voice around their husbands, to act "helpless" and maybe even a little less intelligent than they really were, we are now living in the modern world with modern female rights and advantages. It doesn't mean you have to be serious and not fun to be around, but there are ways to have fun and express yourself that don't involve either of you acting like children. Marilyn Monroe decided that her persona was going to be the "helpless little girl," and many of us still think this is the way to appeal to a man. Although Marilyn was loved by many and was very sexy, according to her close associates, her little-girl persona in her films was very different from her off-screen personality. Even today, many women are still influenced by Marilyn's on-screen persona, to the point where they copy her voice style and childlike innocence, and feel that it's *the* way to "act sexy." Acting less intelligent, less independent, or much younger than you are not only sells yourself short as a woman, it also facilitates more inequality in your relationship. This kind of behavior might be considered sexy by some people, but would you really want to keep that up in a long-term relationship? C'mon! Let's call it what it is: an act. It just doesn't work in a truthful and equal partnership.

We like to call all of these thoughts and actions "subconscious sabotage." You both need to recognize these bad habits and realize what each of you are doing. If you are starting to feel that you are turning into his mother, address it and talk about it with your partner. And likewise, if he feels that he's viewing you as *only* a mother, or even if you suspect he is feeling this way, then you must talk about it. The same thing goes when one or both of you get into the little child mind-set as well. Get it out there in the open! By talking about it, you acknowledge the mistaken way you are feeling. And by sharing those thoughts with each other, you then take away its power to affect you. Then, you both can just ditch all those thoughts and stop the behavior! Consciously throw them away.

Just Get on with It

However easy it is to fall into these kinds of words and thought processes, they aren't going to do anything good for your relationship. And for you women, we don't care if you have one child or ten (or even just a couple of pet Chihuahuas) you are still a woman with many different facets to who you are, beyond just being a wife, mother, or caregiver.

We also don't care what excuses you may have regarding your childhood or your emotional baggage. Let's just keep things simple: don't rehash your entire past. Acknowledge it, take responsibility for it, talk about it briefly, and then, *move on*. Don't get all psycho-analytical about it and beat it to death by analyzing it ad nauseam.

If you spend hours analyzing where these behaviors came from, you start giving them more importance. You don't need loads of therapy for it either! Save yourselves the money. Getting overly cerebral can harm the natural dynamic of your relationship. You both simply end up thinking way too much!

Both of us have spent many years in England, and we took one very important concept away with us: "Just get on with it!" The English don't talk about stuff until they are blue in the face like we Americans sometimes do. They simply say it, recognize it, and then move on. That's it. No endless analyzing! And truly, this is all that is necessary.

Fighting for your sexual relationship is fighting for your relationship as a whole. Make a sign, post it on your fridge, and make it a law: *No baby talk, no kiddie talk, no Mommy talk, and no Daddy talk. Don't do it.* For your relationship to stay hot and healthy, and to last, there needs to be clarity in both of your minds about who you are to each other. You are sexual adults and partners. This is the important element that needs to be present, and remain present, in your minds.

We know it can be difficult to find the right balance between your inner self and your role as mother and as wife. And the same goes for husbands. Your inner core as an individual is made up of many parts of you, and if your inner self is happy, then the rest of life falls into place. Falling in love and having sex was so easy in the beginning, right? Well, let's get back on track by behaving like a man and a woman again. And stop all of this silly talk!

BANNING THE BABY TALK

1 Always use your adult voice when speaking with your partner. Don't allow yourself the habit of falling into the comfy "little baby voice" tone. Whether you have children or not, there are *no excuses*.

2 Once one of you starts using the dreaded "Mommy" or "Daddy," talk about it, acknowledge it, and then throw it away! Remind yourselves that it's impossible to retain a sexual relationship with each other and continue this behavior.

3 If you find yourself overwhelmed at home with chores, children, and so on, and feeling emotionally and physically exhausted, stand up and call time-out! You deserve a break sometimes. Let your partner know your needs—loud and clear.

4 Remember that your household roles and your child-raising roles have nothing to do with your sexual roles. Keep them clearly defined and separate.

5 No matter how much you love your children, remember they are *not* your life. You both are multifaceted human beings. You are adult sexual beings. Embrace all that you are.

Chapter Three

Close the Bathroom Door

*"The secret to a happy marriage is separate bathrooms.
That's essential. Whenever we stay in a hotel we always get
two bedrooms just so we can have an extra bathroom.
It's vital to have your own space so you aren't constantly
in each other's pockets."*

—SIR MICHAEL CAINE, OSCAR–WINNING ACTOR,
 MARRIED TO WIFE SHAKIRA MORE THAN THIRTY-FIVE YEARS
 (*SYDNEY MORNING HERALD*, MARCH 2008)

*"I'm so comfortable with my honey . . . we can even poo
in front of each other!"*

—TIFFANY, AGE 25

LIKE TIFFANY, MANY OF US FALL into the trap of being overly comfortable and open with our partners about every single aspect of our lives. We know that you might enjoy the closeness of being able to share everything together, but what happens to the mystery in the relationship when that occurs? Let's think on this one for a minute and ask ourselves: do we really need to know about each other's bowel movements? We think not. Pooing in front of each other is a definite no-no. That kind of closeness is honestly not necessary unless your partner finds such behavior exciting, but we doubt many of you would have signed up for a lover who was turned on by poo! Now if when we said, "your lover," you were thinking, "Well, he only kind of is at the moment," then you really need to take a look at why that is. And yes, it might have to do with poo! Bathroom behavior can really stink up your sex life, so take heed.

Keep It to Yourselves

Toilet closeness is all part of the downward spiral to lovers becoming roommates. The following couple, Kathy and Steve, both in their late thirties, have been together for ten years. Kathy works in customer service, and Steve is an accountant. Generally, they are a pretty conservative couple . . . except when it comes to their toilet habits.

"The sex is still kind of regular at once a month or so," Kathy told us. She said that the sex is "nice," but nothing like they used to have in the first couple of years. After we shared a girls' night out and a few drinks with Kathy, we began to delve further into toilet topics. When we asked about her and Steve's bathroom habits, this is what she had to say:

"It's so funny with Steve and me. Sometimes he'd do this really *huge* log of a poo he was really proud of. He'd call me into the bathroom and say, 'Look at this, hon, you gotta see the size of this shit I just did!' And I'd run in and we'd both stand there staring down into the toilet in wonderment at the massive thing that just came out of him! We thought it was hilarious! So then after that, it kinda became a bit of a contest . . . to see who could produce the biggest poo. Oh, and then sometimes if we were constipated or something, it became a contest to see who had the smallest, cutest little rabbit pellet of a poo. Yep, we have definitely seen our share of each other's poos!"

Kathy and Steve's behavior is a perfect example of what not to do. It's bad enough if you and your partner share these toilet tales between you, but to share them with friends or family is compounding the problem. For your man to tell a story about you blocking hotel room toilets and boasting to your friends about your "Captain's Log that backed up the Pensacola sewage system" is just plain wrong. This is not the kind of thing you or your partner needs to say and hear. Leave it out. Period.

We wish we didn't have to say this, but if you have diarrhea or constipation or you do a mammoth-size poo, don't share the experience with your lover or anyone you know. Why would you want to do this anyway? What would possess you? If you really are a slightly twisted individual or a comedian who likes toilet humor, and you must share it with someone, then share the story (yes, okay . . . take a digital picture of it if you must) with the people on the Rants & Raves page of Craigslist. Share it anonymously with total strangers that you will never see, know, or speak to, but don't share it with your lover or anyone you know. You and he are supposed to be really hot for each other, right? Then how does any of this behavior increase the desire? It doesn't.

Of course, if you are married, living together, or just spending a lot of time together, it does mean that you will have to use the bathroom when your partner is around. And even though some noises and smells may not be entirely avoidable, care needs to be taken to allow each other some space and distance. You can afford to retain a bit of mystery in this area. Get a fan installed in your bathroom, or get a radio and use it when you are in there. Your partner doesn't need to hear your various farts and plops, now does he? Also, invest in some nice incense or a candle and light it before you start your "business." Even some air freshener will suffice, or at the bare minimum, always have matches at the ready. Lighting a match and wafting it around once you've blown it out is a good, fast way to remove smells.

Now, when you have the urge to go to the bathroom, is it normal for you to say, "Oh, pookie, I need to go have a poopie!" Or, in his case, does he announce that he's "Gonna take a dump?" Not super classy, is it? Let's try to refrain from saying those sorts of things. Instead, just say that you are simply "going to the bathroom" and that you may "be a few minutes or so." And, "please take a message if someone calls or pops by . . . I'll need some alone time." That's it. Don't elaborate. Make it understood that questions do not need to be asked about what you'll be doing in there. It has to be a pact that you and your significant other stick with. Your sexual relationship is more important than being casual about your bathroom etiquette. You wouldn't want to go to the bathroom in front of a new lover—so don't do it in front of your most important lover—your long-term partner.

We all tend to forget about the respect and distance necessary to keep a sexual relationship healthy. It should make no difference whether we've known each other for ten hours or ten years. Don't walk in on each other when you are having this "alone time" in the bathroom. We know it feels funny at first to backtrack and to start being more formal in this area once again, but what do you have to lose? Wouldn't you rather have more hot sex—the kind that makes you feel young, sexy, passionate, and alive—like you did in the past? Stupid question, right? So, have some faith in the process, start creating some distance, and get some mystery back in this area.

It's Time to "Powder Our Nose" Again

We realize, though, that our lives are much more casual these days as compared to life fifty years ago. For instance, can you imagine Clark Gable saying to Carole Lombard that he needed to "take a whizz"? Or likewise, can you imagine Grace Kelly telling Cary Grant that she was going to go "squeeze out a shit"? Not likely. In those days, there was a level of self-respect and a sense of dignity that is sadly lacking in our modern world. These days, everyone likes to hang loose and be casual, but trust us, this is not always a good thing. We need formal boundaries in this area, and looking back to that period is a good place to start. Nowadays when women are out at a restaurant, it's not unusual to hear them say, "I gotta go pee" in front of their lover, their friends, and even new acquaintances. Too many of us are guilty of this behavior, simply because it has become acceptable. But, like calling your spouse "honey," just because everyone does it, doesn't mean that it's right.

Simon and Annabel, both in their early twenties, had been dating for about four months. Both live in New York City and work in the nightclub industry. Simon is a bartender from Manhattan, and Annabel is a waitress, originally from Newcastle, England. They had a lot in common; they loved watching soccer, they were both obsessed with Indian food, and the sex was great. But, unfortunately, they didn't last. Simon tells us why he broke off the relationship:

"When I first met Annabel, we were working at the same nightclub. She was really sexy, really fun, and just easy to be around. At first, I'd notice that she'd say stuff like, 'Oh, hang on, love, I've gotta go have a wettie.' I guess that didn't really bother me too much in the beginning because a lot of people say they have to go have a pee. Also, being that she was originally from Newcastle, I figured that was just her cute Northern English way. But after awhile, she'd comment on what went on every single time she'd go. She'd say stuff like, 'Bloody hell, I really flooded the loo with that gusher. I was bursting!' Or, 'Phew, that pee went on for so long, my piss flaps are tired!' Some people thought it was funny that she'd say things like that. She was so forward about that stuff, it was kind of her way. The problem for me was, she always did it. It didn't matter where we were or what kind of company we were in, she never had any qualms about talking like that. Being from the city and working at a nightclub, I'd figured I'd heard it all anyway, so I kept convincing myself that this was fairly normal nowadays. Especially with English girls claiming to be 'ladettes' now as well (at least that was what she would call herself for some reason). I mean, it's just part of being the modern woman, I guess.

"There was another time that I thought was a bit much too. We had arranged a date for breakfast one Sunday, and we were meeting in the West Village downtown. The minute I saw her, when she was coming out of the subway, she started going on about how sorry she was for being late because she had just gotten her period. She starting telling me, 'Sorry babes, I just got on the rag, and when I woke up this morning there was blood everywhere. It was like bloody World War Three in the bed or something! It had gotten on the mattress cover and even the mattress itself! I had to wash it all off before it left a permanent stain. So, sorry about me being late, hon. Anyway, where do ya' wanna' eat brekkie?' After Annabel told me that story, to be honest, I felt a bit sick. Then when she talked about breakfast in practically the same breath, it just put me off the idea of eating entirely.

"But I think the final statement that really put the nail into the coffin on our relationship was this one time at the club. The manager and all the other bar staff were hanging around waiting for the club to get busy, and she said just out of the blue, 'God, I've got such cramps at the moment—my period is so heavy my tampon is gurgling!' It was so disgusting! And the fact that she shared it with everyone as well . . . it just really put me off her. She was just so crass. She totally grossed me out after that, so much so that I didn't want to have sex with her anymore. So, I made some stupid excuse, and broke it off."

It's true that we are living in a modern world where women are free to do so many things: take the birth control pill, drink and smoke in public, have one-night stands, vote, have a career, even cuss and swear if we want to, amongst many other things. Yes, we have been truly liberated. But does this really give us the go-ahead to be crass and disgusting? To talk about things that really should be private? Whose business is it anyway what goes on with you in the bathroom? Just because you are having sex with someone doesn't mean he has to hear all of your toilet commentaries.

Years ago, the common phrase women would have used for anything having to do with the bathroom was, "Excuse me, I need to go powder my nose." It's sweet, it's feminine, and most important, it's classy. And, even if you do have to actually powder your nose, do you have to do it at the table in front of guests? No. It's just plain tacky. Personal grooming should be just that—personal. Even when it's something as innocent as actually powdering your nose, or reapplying your lipstick, it's not necessary to share it with others. We should embrace some of the good womanly habits and phrases from years ago, and retain a bit of mystery. Remember, privacy is good!

The Sounds of . . . Oh Dear!

Another thing that should be done in private, or at least kept to a minimum, is burping. This applies to both halves in a couple. Granted, it is a necessary bodily function, but it still needs to be done discreetly. Let's think about when you first met and started dating: would either you or he burp in front of one another? Okay, maybe you did a little, but we bet it was quiet and subdued. Or else you did it coyly by putting your hand over your mouth. Our guess is that you made sure it was nearly imperceptible. In fact, we'd be willing to bet that neither of you made a point of letting out the biggest belch known to mankind. And back then, he wasn't trying to belch the national anthem, either. So what has happened since? Do you now have belching contests where the biggest, loudest, longest wins? *Nice.* You've traded your sexual passion for each other for the right to belch and belch loudly! And you've thrown some of your extra artistic talent and innovation in there too. Really? Why would you *do* that?

Okay, you knew we were going to get around to it: farting. Yes, farting offers hours of laughs and amusement: him saying "pull my finger," or farting in bed and then releasing the covers and engulfing you both in the full, concentrated odor of the silent but deadly fart as a "joke." And there's the all-time favorite, farting *on* each other. *Lovely.* Listen, blowing the covers off the bed every morning is not a good thing in a relationship. Nor is drunkenly floating in a crowded hotel pool after a spicy dinner and producing a stream of bubbles from your bottom while shouting, "Look out! Gas attack!" We know it can be fun and funny, but what do you think that's doing to your passion for each other? Share that humor with your friends if you must but not your lover. Here's a challenge: find other ways of being humorous, without resorting to toilet humor.

Sometimes though, we just can't help doing an inadvertent fart. We tried not to. We thought it was going to be a silent one and not smelly (or deadly). But there it is, an audible fart. What do you do? We know that the first time you fart in front of someone new, it's pretty darn embarrassing, right? What do you usually say when this happens? You probably say, "Oh, excuse me." This is good! This is the right reaction. Keep on behaving this way, whether you're with a stranger or your partner of thirty years. On the other hand, if it's just a little "poot" you should probably just ignore it or cough. But if you've already started down the oh-so-humorous road of fart games, stop immediately, and start doing the right thing. Be polite, respectful, and dignified. You won't regret it.

Tinkle Tinkle

This behavior modification also applies to peeing. Pee on your own, ladies! Close that bathroom door! He doesn't need to see you peeing or wiping. This is not a good vision, no matter how attractive you try to appear when you perform this function. And likewise, you don't have to stand there watching urine coming out of his penis while talking about the shopping list! Looking at his penis should be a turn on, right? Watch his penis when you're having intercourse, when you're sucking on it, or when you're playing with it, but don't stare at it when he's peeing. How is that going to turn you on?

We know at this point you may be thinking that it's just unrealistic not to do something as simple and commonplace as peeing in front of each other. And we know that you're thinking, *But it's not really gross like pooing or farting, right?* True. But, here's the thing: it's not the peeing once or twice in front of each other that does the damage to your sexual relationship. It's the ongoing daily performance of bathroom bodily functions that slowly but surely kills the frisson and the mystery you once had. Wouldn't you like to get that frisson back? Then stop going to the bathroom in front of each other! Do you really think you'll miss the vision of him "taking a dump," "dropping the kids off at the pool," or "taking the Browns to the Super Bowl?" And, do you really need to watch him peeing and then flicking the last drops off the end of his penis? We don't think so. It's time to put some mystery back in the relationship and keep the bad habits out.

Hide the Gory Details

Mystery also applies when riding that scarlet wave. Do not insert or pull out bloody tampons in front of your man! His penis or tongue goes in there, remember? Does he want to see some cotton thingy dripping with blood coming out of there? We doubt it. And the same applies to pads and panty liners. Most guys get pretty grossed out simply watching a maxipad commercial when the blue liquid is poured on to the pad. So how much worse is it for him to see the real thing all soaked and matted on a pad? A lot worse! Unless you really do want to gross him out, we think it's best to keep it private. We guarantee that your guy does not want to see the full glory of day two of your period, or the brownish remnants of the last day either! He doesn't want to see it, and he doesn't want to hear about it either. And for God's sake, do not chase him around the room scaring him with your bloody tampon because you think it's funny! It might be funny for you, but he's gonna have nightmares. Let's be honest here, even we don't find it pleasurable viewing. So why share it?

Flush and Forget

We realize, however, that there can be unfortunate times when sharing an unseemly moment together is totally unavoidable. Honeymooners Sarah and Mark, both in their late twenties, had such an experience. After a blissful few days in Puerta Vallarta, Mexico, they ended up with a bad case of Montezuma's revenge. Something as unpredictable as diarrhea can still be private even if you have it simultaneously—that is, if you have the luxury of separate bathrooms like Michael Caine and his wife. But if you have only one bathroom, as in Sarah and Mark's case during their honeymoon, this can pose a problem. Sarah recalls their experience:

"We had this great meal at a fabulous restaurant in the main part of town. The food was superb, as were the blended margaritas. I remember we kept commenting to each other with every bite and sip that it was our best meal there yet! Well, it turned out to be too good to be true. We woke up the next day feeling awful. Both Mark and I had really bad diarrhea. And I'm not talking about mild diarrhea that you can kind of control. And worse, we both *had* to go at exactly the same time! But, with only one toilet in the room, one of us had to perch on the sink and the other on the toilet. We were only two feet from each other during the entire incident. Throughout the day it would keep happening, and we ended up taking turns on who got the toilet and who got the sink. We laughed about the ridiculousness of it at the time, but really it was pretty disgusting!"

Mark and Sarah's story is probably the worst-case bathroom scenario a couple can experience. You and your partner may never experience this particular kind of unwanted intimacy and mucho embarrassment, but if you do suffer an experience like Mark and Sarah's, it doesn't need to do permanent damage to your sexual attraction for each other. Here's what needs to be done after something like that: Put it behind you! Don't continue to reminisce about it or think of your loved one squatting over the sink. However tempting it is to share this "hilarious experience" with each other or with friends, don't retell the story. Every time you relive that experience, you chip away at the sexual tension between you. Just forget about it, and put it into the far reaches of your mind. It was an incident you shared together, however unfortunate, and now you need to move on with dignity. Respect and dignity are always key.

The Offensive Super Bowl

Lack of respect certainly played a major part in the demise of the following couple, Amanda and Chris. They were both in their midthirties and had been living together for eight years. They had an online business they ran together and spent nearly all of their time with one another. We talked to Amanda and asked her why she had split with her partner, Chris, when everyone thought they were such a fabulous couple. They had so much in common and loved spending time together, but when it came to toilet issues, it was clear that mutual respect had fallen by the wayside. Amanda confided to us one afternoon:

"When I first met Chris, I thought he was the most handsome man I had ever seen, in person or in the movies. He was like a cross between George Clooney and Brad Pitt, with his jet-black hair, piercing blue eyes, and sexy dimples. I couldn't believe it when he asked me for my number! The strange thing was that even though I worshiped the way he looked, my sexual desire for him diminished pretty quickly. It was after Chris started farting in front of me and leaving the bathroom door open whenever he sat on the toilet that our sex life took a big turn for the worse. He literally didn't care what disgusting thing I saw him do—whether it was sitting on the toilet and farting, cutting his nose hairs, picking his toes on the coffee table, or scratching his balls all day long. Sometimes he would show me the inside of his jogging shorts and he'd say, 'Look honey, I was jogging so hard that I had the Hershey squirts in my shorts, and I didn't even know it!' I told him to stop being so disgusting, but he'd just laugh and said I was being uptight. I was so turned off that we only had sex about once a month and even then I only did it because he kept begging me. I kept trying to get him to cut out his vile habits, but I think he just didn't care.

"The straw that broke the camel's back, so to speak, happened one Sunday afternoon. Chris was sitting on the toilet with the door open and leaning forward so he could still see the football game on the living room TV. I walked by and Chris said, 'Isn't this great? I can take a shit and still watch the game at the same time!' Then to my horror, he spread his legs apart and lifted his rear off the toilet! He was like a proud kid wanting to show me his 'creation.' I screamed, 'Chris, that's it! Don't *ever* show me something like that again!' I then ran to the bedroom, feeling sick to my stomach.

"Looking back on that incident, I think it had a devastating effect on my image of Chris as a sexual partner. I could never get that vision out of my head of him smiling and lifting his rear off the toilet. Even though he was still just as handsome, the thought of having sex with him went completely out of my head that afternoon and never came back. That was the trouble with seeing Chris in that state, it was just impossible to erase that picture from my mind."

The fact that Chris took such glee in sharing these things with Amanda was just plain wrong. Obviously, Chris had lost respect in the relationship—not only respect for Amanda but also for himself. The reason Amanda was so angry wasn't just that these incidents occurred but that Chris took such pleasure in sharing them. An unavoidable situation like Mark and Sarah's "Montezuma incident" is forgivable and forgettable, simply because it was purely unintentional. But Chris's behavior toward Amanda was a completely different situation. It *was* avoidable. And worse, it was a pattern of boorish behavior, bordering on abuse. This all led to Amanda's unhappiness, resentment, and eventually the breakup of their relationship. Some of you might think this scenario is hilarious, picturing a guy with a huge poop hanging out of his bottom. But, hilarity aside, a couple can't survive this kind of behavior. Chris and Amanda are no longer the fabulous, happy couple they were, and this is a tragedy. They might still be together today, if only some of these issues had been addressed.

The Toilet Seat and the Damage Done

Moving on from the disgusting to the simply annoying: even repeating a simple action such as leaving the toilet seat up can do damage to a relationship. It may seem like a silly request, but when it comes to the toilet, it is important to close the lid. This is just basic courtesy and shouldn't be considered a huge effort. It's better romantically, aromatically, and even aesthetically. It also shows you have consideration and respect for your partner.

According to the principles of feng shui, by leaving the toilet lid up, you not only flush away the contents of whatever was formally in you but also all the good energy in your home. So, on many different levels, it's always a great idea to put the seat and the lid down. Guys, this means you! You are no longer allowed to flip everything up, whip it out, pee, shake it off, and then leave, and not wash your hands. It may seem trivial to you but the difference it will make to your partner is massive. Just think about all the times you left the seat up. How annoying do you think it gets for her? How much more annoyed and resentful do you think she feels when you continue to do it again and again? Resentment can start with small, seemingly insignificant things, but over time, it can build up and become a huge mountain of anger.

From the disgusting incident that Amanda experienced with Chris to the seemingly innocuous habit of leaving the toilet seat up, all of these acts can do a huge amount of damage to a relationship. Repetition of these acts can be the difference between a happy marriage and divorce. It is often the buildup of the little things that can totally break down the relationship. We've all been guilty of having huge fights with our partners about things that might seem trivial: a toilet seat left up, drops of urine on the floor, or even just squeezing the toothpaste the "wrong" way. Respect for your lovers means listening to them, and taking their requests seriously. Obviously if one partner is naturally messier than the other, care needs to be taken to reach a compromise where both sides feel comfortable and don't harbor any resentment.

There are plenty of other little things that we're sure many of you do in front of each other, both in and out of the bathroom, that can cause problems. Things such as cutting your toenails, picking the dead skin off your feet (while sitting at the breakfast table!), picking your nose, squeezing zits, shaving your pubes, trimming your nose hair, flossing, spitting (in all its full-phlegmy glory), putting on those green face masks . . . we could go on and on. But here's what you need to ask yourself, "Would I be doing this in front of someone I have just met?" If the answer is no, then common sense dictates you shouldn't be doing it in front of your partner now either. It's all a respect thing. Respect and dignity are requirements, not options.

Now we know that men especially can get lazy in these areas. They may accuse us women of being uptight when we ask them to change their bathroom habits. But here is what you want to impress upon him: Does he want to have more and better sex? Does he want you to be ready, willing, and excited to "have" him? Or is having a shit and picking his nose in front of you more important to him than having sex with you? When you put it to him like that, he will see the connection, and, thankfully, most men will always take the road of more sex! Remind him playfully of this if he starts down that icky road again. Don't let him think you're a nag. Instead, just simply say something along the lines of, "Hey baby, do you want to fuck me later? Then close that door, and I'll be here waiting for you!"

Remember that most men and women have never made the connection between an open bathroom–door policy and little or no sex. This is why we need to remind each other that bathroom etiquette is not just being polite with one another; it's integral to saving your sex life and saving your relationship as a whole.

Not Always a Spectator Sport

This next subject isn't a toilet topic per se, but it is an important thing to consider. Having a baby and bringing a new life into the world is a beautiful and meaningful experience. If your partner wants to be there with you and you are happy to have him there, then by all means share that together. This can bring a new, deeper, and even more spiritual bond to your relationship. That said, having a baby can also be a bit of a gory experience. There is the water breaking, the blood, the mucus, the possible bowel movement when you are in midpush . . . and when the baby is crowning, it is almost surreal. And gore doesn't begin to describe the afterbirth, the possible tearing, and following that, the stitching up of the area.

One couple shared their story with us. Cindy and Dean, both in their early thirties, had just experienced the birth of their son, a whopping ten-pound baby! Unfortunately, Cindy tore quite badly when the child's head was crowning. Once the baby was calm and the afterbirth had been expelled, the doctor started getting ready to sew up Cindy's torn vagina. It was at that point that Dean made the mistake of looking more closely at the area. He saw that it looked nothing like what a vagina normally looks like. Instead, he said it looked like a cross between, "a pile of raw ground beef and a bizarre biological lab experiment." Looking at the doctor in horror, Dean said, "How in the hell are you going to fix *that*?" Of course the good doctor did repair the damage, but the vision of his wife's torn, raw-looking vagina has never left his mind. Now each time the opportunity for oral sex presents itself, Dean told us that his recurring vision of the "ground beef" is a big turnoff, and the oral sex, if it happens at all, has become perfunctory, not fun.

It's important with the birth of a child to talk about what you would like to experience together and what really isn't necessary. It might be that in some cases, the experience needs to be had with the man up by the woman's face, rather than staring intently at his wife's vagina. All the aspects of the birth need to be discussed and thought out ahead of time. This way you can both feel pretty confident that nothing will scar your memory of this wondrous event.

Having a baby is a beautiful thing and having that experience together shouldn't be denied. But here's the important thing to remember: What one should focus on is the memory of bringing that beautiful baby into the world. Don't focus on the blood, the afterbirth, and the state of the vagina immediately after the birth. Put that part of it out of your mind and move on.

From the seemingly insignificant act of urinating in front of each other, to the momentous event of bringing a new life into the world, couples need to understand their boundaries and stick to them. We all need to continually treat our partners with consideration and offer privacy when necessary. It is never good for you and your partner to be comfortable going to the bathroom in front of each other. You aren't *supposed* to be comfortable doing these things in front of other people. If you have gone too far down that road, just turn around and start afresh. Remember: resentment and anger can rear their ugly heads when a partner suggests stopping this kind of behavior and it goes unheeded. It's all about mutual respect. Never forget that each time you continue to perform toilet acts in front of each other, there will be a slow ebbing away of your relationship—a transformation from lovers to just friends.

Imagine Rodin, the famous sculptor, has just finished his masterpiece of you and your lover. It's called "The Lovers," of course. He's depicted you and your partner in the early stages of your relationship, together in a passionate embrace. Every time you and your lover disregard the boundaries of bathroom behavior, Rodin chisels away a little more of the passion and mystery between you. Every day, more and more is being chipped away, and sadly, this once-beautiful sculpture is now unrecognizable. But what a shame, because you and your lover were pretty darn fabulous when you were passionate. Let's try to keep it that way.

AVOID BEING HIS BATHROOM BUDDY

1   Keep those bathroom necessities to yourself. Intimacy in the bedroom: good. Intimacy in the bathroom: bad. Privacy is king.

2   Don't embellish things like burping, farting, and other audible bodily functions. However "funny" you think it is, it's not. It's damaging to your sexual desire for one another.

3   When unpleasant things happen that are accidental or unavoidable, simply say, "Excuse me," and move on. Don't continue to relive embarrassing moments or talk about them, either to each other or to friends.

4   Always respect your partner's boundaries and listen to their concerns. Your idea of messy and his idea of messy might be very different. You both need to compromise.

5   Even the most trivial habits, repeated often enough, can lead to less sexual desire and possible resentment. Sex and resentment are never good bed partners!

Chapter Four

Look into His Eyes

*"This guy I am seeing. . . we have the most intimate sex.
It is unworldly. He holds my face and looks into my eyes the
entire time. He touches my lips. He stares at my naked body
and goes about everything really slow. We have sessions that last
like six hours of touching and fondling, etc. He cuddles all
night. I awake to him rubbing my hands or touching my hair.
It is the most intimate experience ever in my life."*

—SUSAN, AGE 36

*"I still love it when my husband looks into my eyes.
It reminds me why I love him."*

—RHONDA, AGE 53

WHEN YOU FIRST GOT TOGETHER with your partner, you
talked like crazy just wanting to know all about each other, right?
But let's think back on that first meeting and that very moment

before you actually spoke. Maybe it all started with a lingering look at each other from across a room, just a moment longer than necessary. Maybe he spotted you or you spotted him first. But let's think about the impact of that first moment . . . when your eyes met. Was it verbal? Nope. Or, even if your first meeting *was* verbal and you were introduced by a mutual friend or acquaintance, our guess is that there was that moment—that indefinable moment— when you looked into each other's eyes and you both knew you were interested. And later, there was that first date or that first more private conversation, and inevitably, those sexually charged moments when you'd silently look into each other's eyes. What were your thoughts back then? We'd be willing to bet you were thinking about his lips and how you hoped he'd grab you and start kissing you, right then and there. Or even how it would be to have him on top of you while passionately making love. We bet there wasn't a lot of verbalizing those thoughts to him just then. It's not like you would immediately tell him exactly everything you were thinking —he's a guy you had just met! Whether you both were thinking about ripping each others clothes off or quietly gazing into each other's eyes over a glass of wine—the truth is that you both felt a primal attraction to each other that didn't need to be put into words.

Now that we've taken you back to those thoughts and feelings in the early days of your relationship, we bet you are thinking, *Well, that is pretty much gone . . . so now what? I still love him but where is that spark?* Well, you really can get that feeling back! Hopefully at this point, you fully understand the importance of not calling each other silly pet names, and you have also banished the baby talk and changed your bathroom habits, too. Now that you've swept out all of that "verbal rubbish" that was impeding your sex life in the past, you've got a fresh start. You can explore the other ways of communicating that you have probably forgotten—like those sexually charged glances into each other's eyes when you first met. But how do you do that? Where do you start?

Well, the best place to begin is to look into each other's eyes. It is our most basic form of communication and the most powerful. Sometimes we're so busy with our lives that we've forgotten how important that silent connection can be between a couple—that special look and touch that we can give each other throughout the day that signals to our partners that we're very happy and grateful to be their lovers. Our lives can be so hectic that we can go *weeks* without even stopping to really look into each other's eyes. Most couples don't see each other during the day—when both partners are working or running the household. And when they are at home together at night, they eat dinner watching the evening news before they run around the house doing chores and taking care of the kids, only to fall asleep the minute their heads hit the pillow. This is when the simple, physical connection between a couple can get lost.

The eyes can be the most intimate and one of the sexiest ways to communicate with your lover. They are not only the window to our souls, but also the window to our sexuality. Get close, and *look* at your partner—really look into his eyes every day for at least a few minutes. Sometimes communicating has nothing to do with words at all. It's the way we look at one another, the way we brush our hand across our partner's neck, or the way we hold hands tightly in a crowded room. Not talking gives us a chance to stop and take a breath and actually *experience* each other, whether you are both in bed, sitting across the dining table, or even standing across the room at a party. We can't stress enough how important it is for your relationship to do this. Let your souls connect with that look. You don't need to say a word.

We need a little mystery to feel sexy with our partner as well, and always verbalizing everything is not mysterious or sexy. Remember when the strong, silent type was considered sexy? Well, it still is, for men and for women. Sex can be very visual. This is why simply letting your eyes do the talking for you, without a lot of chatter, can create a sexually charged atmosphere. Silence gives both of you a chance to create a fantasy between you. Silence can build tension, and tension builds lust.

Looking at each other in or out of bed is a great way to slow things down and to reacquaint yourself with the person you're with every night. It gives the sexual side of your brain a chance to breathe a little, something we don't do often enough. This will also allow your mind a chance to retreat from the day and all of its problems and enjoy a blissful moment or two of sexual fantasy. Sex is much more in the mind than we realize; it's also sometimes more of a fantasy play than a reality play. We need to take that time to allow our intimate nonverbal communication to jump-start our mental fantasies once again. For instance, whether your fantasy is that you and your husband are in a different place or you are playing roles in your head that you are different people in a sexy situation, you need to give your minds that chance to explore and be creative. This is when sex can have limitless possibilities and fun. The sky is the limit!

There is nothing wrong with a little fantasizing sometimes.

Although the ubiquitous date night that you read about in many self-help books is certainly not the panacea that the so-called experts contend it is, it does have one good quality. When you are on a date with your husband and sitting at a restaurant enjoying that first glass of wine, you do look into each other's eyes—often more than you did all week. There's no television to stare at, no newspapers to bury your head into, and no children or other adults vying for your attention. It's just you and your man acknowledging your bond together. And it's that acknowledgment of each other as a man and a woman that is so stimulating and powerful. Much more effective than a thousand words about your wants and needs.

Even during everyday moments you can create that spark of sexuality between you. For instance, when you have both come back from the supermarket and are putting away the groceries, take a moment to turn to him—not speaking a word—look into his eyes, and just kiss him slowly and softly. Keep doing that for a moment or two. It's amazing how easily you both can be transported to a place where you feel sexual. You just have to take the time to let yourselves really look at each other.

Allowing yourselves just a few minutes a day to visually connect with one another is often all it takes to keep the sexual fires burning in a long-term relationship. It can be as simple as an exchange during your day together, letting each other know that you look forward to being in bed together later.

Staring at the Wrong Box

David and Nicole, who have been married two years, have experienced the impact that a daytime visual connection can have on a couple. Nicole explained to us one afternoon:

"Even though we've only been married a couple of years, I recently noticed that we had already lost a lot of steam in the bedroom. We had gone from doing it about every other day to only about once a week. I started to panic because I thought, *Oh God, if we only feel like having sex once a week* now, *what's it going to be like in ten years?* And not only was the sex more infrequent, but it had become kind of routine as well. A girlfriend of mine recommended that I get some sex toys, and that kind of worked to heat things up for a couple of weeks, but it didn't last that long and soon we were back to where we were.

"Looking back on our marriage, I became aware that the sex between us started to wane when we started watching TV during dinner. We both have really busy jobs—we're both hospital nurses—so when we come home, we do like to veg out. I thought about it, though, and I realized that those conversations we used to have over dinner, looking at each other across the table, were what really kept us connected during our first year together. We work twelve-hour shifts, and there isn't always a lot of time to spend together, but the TV seemed to eat up any awake time that we had. The problem was that not only would we watch TV during dinner, but then we would somehow just leave it on until we went to bed. We hardly even talked to each other anymore, let alone looked at each other!

"So I said to David one day that I thought we should stop watching TV during dinner and take some time to really talk again. At first it was hard because I could tell that he missed the news, especially sports, and that hurt my feelings. But I was insistent about it. I told him that we could both watch TV after dinner, but that dinner was a time of talking and connecting with each other. And it really did work! After a couple of weeks, I noticed the change that happened just because we were once again looking at each other, instead of the TV set. And it led to other rituals, too—like every couple of days we go out to the yard and sip some wine before dinner and just hold hands and talk. We've started to take walks after dinner too, which has been great for us as a couple. It feels really romantic doing something simple like walking around the block at night. The funny thing is, the less we watched TV, the less we felt like watching it. I'd much rather look at my husband than some stupid TV show!"

We asked Nicole how this change in routine had affected their sex life:

"It's been great. We're nearly back to where we were in the beginning of the relationship. The sex is not only more often, but hotter too! It's weird the difference it makes spending some time with each other without a lot of distractions. Just looking into each other's eyes and making the time only for each other have both made a huge difference. I feel like we've got our connection back."

As with David and Nicole, sometimes just a small change in a daily routine can make a huge difference in a couple's sexual connection. The seemingly harmless practice of watching TV during dinner can have many repercussions that couples don't realize until they stop the behavior. What's important to learn here is that the simple act of looking at one another and really focusing on each other can be extremely powerful. Keeping the world and its many distractions at bay, and taking a few minutes to look into your partner's eyes and reconnect is essential for a healthy relationship and a strong sexual bond.

The sexual tension that develops from that nonverbal communication helps bring back those great encounters that you remember from the beginning of your relationship. It also provides that bit of mystery again. Unfortunately in our modern world, because we are constantly talking on the cell phone, Twittering, Facebooking, e-mailing, and texting, we have gotten into the bad habit of always letting everyone know what our latest thought is, no matter how banal it might be. This is not good with a sexual partner because it leaves no room for mystery. Don't always tell him every thought that comes into your head—leave a little out for him to wonder about. Just like he doesn't need to know everything about your bathroom habits, he also doesn't need to know every single thought that crosses your mind during the day.

When your partner thinks *Wow, I can't really figure her out!* that's when he wants to have sex with you. When your partner thinks you are a complex person, that's when he thinks you're sexy. A little silence at the right time can add that element of mystery and suspense. This doesn't mean that you are always silent, of course. What it means is that you don't always blurt out everything that is on your mind at every moment . . . just like when you were first together.

So, don't go to bed talking about how you're going to pay the bills this month, what an irritating person your boss is, or how you really didn't like the dessert your friend served at the latest Bunco gathering. These are conversations that should be over by the time you go to bed! Have these kinds of talks in the living room or in the kitchen—anywhere but in the bedroom.

Don't Ask, Don't Tell

What so many self-help books don't seem to address is that putting everything into words is not always a good thing. This can actually do more damage than good, especially to a couple's sex life. Many books advise women and men to verbalize all of their sexual desires (usually referred to as "intimacy needs") and to do this either in bed or over a cup of coffee at the kitchen table, kind of like an at-home therapy session or a business meeting with your husband—not very sexy at all! And really, not all things have to be acutely analyzed and verbalized, especially when it comes to your sexual selves. You're certainly not going to want to rip each other's clothes off after one of these talks! We can't think of a more doomed way to try to improve your sex life. Sex works when it's natural, nonintellectual, and fun. The following story is a good example of one couple who verbalized and negotiated the sex right out of their relationship.

Gabriella and Dane were high-school sweethearts, and ended up getting married only a few years after graduation. Gabriella tells us her story:

"Initially, like so many couples the sex was great in the beginning. When we first got together, we hadn't talked about sex. We would just do it and not talk. It was fun and passionate and spontaneous. But after being married a short time, things started getting kind of routine and we weren't really connecting sexually anymore. As time went on, we started having less and less sex, and I felt I should try to do something about it. So, I got this self-help book that told me the way to fix our sex life was to discuss all of our sexual needs with each other—even to the point of writing down lists of what we wanted in bed. Dane and I would have several discussions about those needs and desires. It's probably more my fault that I pushed this upon us. I would always want to discuss and analyze every little aspect of our sex life. I guess I had this romanticized view of what a marriage should be—that we should know every single thing about each other and every thought. Like, to be properly joined, we must know it all. But the funny thing is, talking about it didn't make our sex life any better. It actually made it much worse! It totally dried up all of the passion and spontaneity we had in the beginning. And, because we knew every thought and every desire, it started feeling awkward to have sex at all! It just wasn't fun anymore. There was no mystery or excitement left. It had all been talked away. In the end, we stopped having sex entirely, and last year, after spending seven years together, we finally broke up. It just seems like a waste to me now. I know in my future relationships, I'm not going to verbalize every little thing."

In the fifties and sixties, when no one talked about what turned them on in bed or even about sex at all, verbalizing everything made sense because it needed to be done. Back then, sex was thought of as something mainly for the man, to give him pleasure and to satisfy his physical desires. If the woman happened to have an orgasm along the way, that was great, but it certainly wasn't the focus of the exercise. Even in the seventies, talking about sex with your partner was still new, and many women would say that their husband was a "big dummy" when it came to knowing what to do with a woman's clitoris. Back then, the school of thought that men needed to be taught what to do in bed made sense. But not now.

After decades of sex talk, sex movies, sex books, and magazine articles, every known mechanical thing involved when two people come together is known by pretty much *everyone*. Even magazines for teenagers talk about "The latest fifty sex tricks" to try out on your partner. And yes, these little tricks are extremely explicit!

It may sound shocking to say, but nowadays your man probably doesn't need to be told what to do in bed. Chances are he knows very well what turns a woman on. So giving him a list of your desires or needs is just going to make him feel pressured and won't add to the experience. The same also goes for you when he tells you all the things he wants you to do to him. It becomes an analytical "step one, step two, step three" experience. It's certainly organized and efficient, but definitely not sexy. Sex shouldn't be like following an Ikea instruction manual—you're supposed to be having fun, not assembling a *Klingsbo* side table!

Another thing to remember is that your man may have the kind of job where people are telling him what to do all day long. Does he really want to hear instructions from you regarding sex after a long day at work? Isn't that going to make him feel that sex is another chore—another place where he's got to follow orders? Talk about neutering your man—that is the surefire way!

Don't Be a Foreman!

When you give your partner instructions in bed, like "I'd really like oral sex right now . . . no, no, not like that . . . like this," it's not only a major mood killer, but it also sets up the scenario where your partner might say no. He might not feel like doing what you're asking him to do at that moment. This does happen, and you have to expect that sometimes. Just because you ask him for oral sex doesn't mean that he wants to dive in at that moment and go to work. But because you've asked him, you're going to feel rejected if he answers no. This is when anger and resentment can easily rear their ugly heads in the bedroom.

The difference in using a more primal and nonverbal approach is that he can move on to something else if he doesn't feel like doing what you're suggesting. This way, it won't seem like a rejection to you. A nonverbal approach to this scenario would be if you gently pushed his head downward, for example. Or, another way would be to lie in bed and make sure he gets a good look at you below the waist, while giving him a very inviting look. This is much more sexually stimulating for both of you anyway.

Shut Up and Do It!

Sex should be the act of two people expressing themselves in bed, physically, instead of having a discussion about each other's "intimacy needs." This doesn't mean you stop communicating. Emotionally, you need to have great communication. But as much as we would like to think otherwise, sex is just plain hotter when we don't spend those precious times in bed getting all cerebral about it. The atmosphere needs to be sexually charged for you both to feel sexually motivated. Any talk that does happen, should be words that sound sexy, not words that sound like they came out of a session at the therapist's office. This can happen by connecting to each other with your eyes and your physical selves, and leaving the therapy-type stuff out. Obviously if there are things between you that are continually sexually awkward, then you do need to discuss them, get them out in the open, and then once said, stop! Don't beat the discussion to death. Get out of your heads and let the primal, visual, simple nonverbal communication take over.

Words that you *do* use in bed should also not remind your partner of all the other things we say to each other during the day either; things that, let's be honest, may also irritate the hell out of us about each other. For instance, if you were to say something like, "oh, hon . . . I really wish you'd suck on my nipples more often"—isn't that going to remind him that just ten minutes earlier you said, "oh, hon . . . I really wish you'd clean around the toilet more often"? Or, when you bring up some of the mundane items of the day like, "oh, sweetie . . . did you remember to make that dentist appointment today?"—while your husband is on top of you—don't you think that is going to totally ruin the mood? In both these instances, you can pretty much guarantee that the language you use will *not* keep both of you in the moment. While it's true that words can facilitate sex, and words can maybe move things forward—the wrong words and the wrong intonation are not worth the risk of ruining the mood.

Some bedroom dialogue can also make a partner feel guilty. And guilt and sex never mix well. When you ask your husband to perform in a certain way, isn't that going to make him feel guilty that you had to ask? And that maybe he hasn't been touching you as much as he should be? You might get the result you want, but he'll be doing it because he feels guilty, not because he was in a frame of mind where he actually wanted to do it. Too much talk can lead to more guilt and less sex. But a little silence can transport you and your partner to places in your minds and bodies that you haven't experienced in quite a while. And when sex does happen, it will happen naturally and freely for a change.

Initially, everything happened because you were crazy in lust for each other. You were idealized versions of yourselves when you met and first made love. Now that you actually know your partner, including all of his insecurities and his bad habits, you may think that early feeling of lust is simply impossible now. But it isn't! Something will happen in the silence, trust us. It will be a step toward the original sexual tension and mystery that you enjoyed in the first stages of your romance.

Silence Is an Aphrodisiac

The following story of Jane and her husband, Kyle, illustrates the kind of impact that a little silence can have in your bedroom. Jane kept buying new lingerie outfits with the hope of turning on her husband, Kyle. Nothing seemed to rekindle the kind of passion they had in the beginning, she told us after a couple of cocktails. They had been married for eight years and although they still had sex about twice a month, it didn't have the passion of the first couple of years. Kyle is an actor and often has to be away from home for several days or weeks at a time. Jane, a former model, told us that one of the exciting things about his job is the anticipation and sexual tension that would build up for each of them after they had been apart for some time. Sadly, this kind of sexual tension started to wane recently, and all the sexy outfits she bought didn't seem to make a bit of difference:

"Every time Kyle would come home from a job I would wear a sexy new outfit from Victoria's Secret, but he barely reacted at all. Sometimes he would say something like 'nice outfit,' but that was about it. But one night, things were different. I wore a hot new outfit, and he went totally nuts. We had sex for at least two hours, it was even better than when we were on our honeymoon! And I don't think it was just the outfit."

So we asked Jane, what was so different on that night compared to all of the other nights?

"Well, I came out of the bathroom wearing a sexy bra and panties, and I just walked around the house doing odds and ends. But I didn't say anything about the way I looked like I had done before. In the past, whenever I would try on something sexy, whether it was new panties or a new dress, I would always look to Kyle for some kind of compliment. I would usually say something like, 'Don't I look cute, honey?' Or 'Not bad for a thirty-eight-year-old, huh?' But that night, I didn't say a word. I just gave him some long lingering looks and continued doing what I was doing. I walked around the house a little, sat on the bed, and put a little polish on my toes . . . all the while giving him little knowing glances. But I didn't say anything about the way I looked. In fact, I didn't say much at all. I didn't feel like I needed to say anything. I was just doing my own thing, and conveying with my eyes that I was feeling sexy and I wanted him. And that's when he went nuts. He didn't even wait for my nails to dry!"

The key here is that Jane let her eyes and her body language do the talking for her, and this let Kyle use his imagination for a change. She gave his imagination a chance to work, instead of telling him what he should be thinking when he looked at her. To a man, a woman wearing lingerie and asking for a compliment might as well be fully clothed. It's still the same wife, just in a costume—rather than a sexy, enigmatic creature that the husband can't quite figure out. But a wife in sexy lingerie feeling confident, attractive, and self-possessed is a whole different person to a man. This is a woman that intrigues him. A woman he needs to conquer!

When you say to your husband "Don't I look great in this dress?" or "Don't I look great in this new bra?" you haven't given him the chance to think it himself. (If he never gives you a compliment, however, that *is* something you do need to address.) Prompting him to compliment you could also make him feel guilty that he didn't say it in the first place. And as we said earlier, guilt and sex do not mix well. So don't fish for compliments or sexual fulfillment from your husband. Let it happen naturally.

What Jane's story illustrates is that when you let the mood of the evening happen naturally, you will get a better result. Instead of trying to instigate the mood, let your partner come to you naturally by expressing your inner sexuality. Try to let your fantasies run wild, and behave with your husband as if he's someone you've just met and have agreed to have a night of passionate sex with before you both go back to your everyday lives.

The Ultimate Intimate Connection

Since this chapter is about looking into your partner's eyes, we thought we'd mention one of the most intimate times to try it—

when he's inside you. Yes, during sex: when he's on top of you and your faces are inches apart and you feel all of him inside your body as you both move together in perfect harmony. Have you ever tried opening your eyes at a moment like this? We know that it can sometimes be easier to get your head in an erotic place when you have your eyes closed—most of us masturbate that way, so it's hard to break that habit. But try it sometime, even if just for a few seconds. You may experience a sexual and emotional jolt when you do it—something that you won't forget.

Joy and Rick, both in their late twenties, have been together a couple of years. Although they still live in separate apartments, they sleep together several nights a week. Their sex life is still very fulfilling for both of them. Joy thought she had experienced everything when it comes to sex, until the night she caught Rick looking at her:

"Rick and I have a great sex life, much better than any boyfriends I have ever been with. I never really thought of opening my eyes during sex, but now that I think back on it, it used to bother me when I'd be on top of a man and I'd look down and his eyes would be closed and it would look like he was in a far-off place. But I usually have my eyes closed, so I never gave it too much thought.

"Until one night, when Rick and I were having really slow, almost tantriclike, sex. He was moving really slowly and sensually, and I was too. That's what I love about the way we're so sexually compatible—we both sometimes like to stop and just really feel each other. I've never been the kind of girl that wants a guy to do it superfast all the time. Anyway, Rick was on top of me and for some reason I happened to open my eyes and look up and Rick was staring into my eyes at just that moment. It was the most erotic and bonding moment I had ever experienced. I never really looked into a partner's eyes during sex before, and certainly not at a supersensual moment like that. He continued to move slowly and even more deeply inside me, never taking his gaze off me. It was like he was boring into me with everything he had—his eyes, his penis, his soul. I can't even describe it—but it was very powerful. I had never experienced that kind of closeness with a man. I felt so bonded to him after that night, like I never felt toward a man before. Now we don't do it every time we have sex, but when it does happen it's still like an electric jolt going through my body!"

As Joy explained, looking into each other's eyes during sex doesn't have to be done all the time. Women do have to get their heads in an erotic place, and usually that means closing their eyes. And the same goes for men, too. But try opening them and staring at your partner every once in a while. What we've learned from the men we've spoken with is that they like to be looked at during sex, too. It makes them feel like you're really thinking of them, and not closing your eyes and thinking of Brad Pitt instead. They feel appreciated. It will probably bring you even closer together than you ever could have anticipated. Isn't it amazing how much can be said without actually saying a word?

Lay, Lady, Lay

The following couple, Sam and Arlene, are an example of great early nonverbal communication that somehow got lost along the way. Arlene, fifty-one years old, has been happily married to Sam for thirty years:

"When Sam wants to have sex with me, it is usually only just once a month or so. He usually says something like, 'Hey there, feel like a little pokey-pokey tonight?' which is okay, but not the way it was in the beginning. I remember one of the most erotic things that he would do in the beginning was to surprise me by turning off the lights in the bedroom and laying there naked. It was really sexy because it was unexpected and he didn't say anything. We would be doing dishes and getting the kids in bed—that kind of thing—and he would go to the bedroom and turn off all the lights and wait for me. When I would enter the bedroom he wouldn't say a word—it would be so dark that I couldn't even see him. I loved the fact that he would take control like that. I would usually strip off all my clothes and lay next to him and we would lay there in silence. It was really sexy because we didn't know what would happen next. Sometimes I would reach over and start touching his penis, sometimes we would just start kissing and stroking each other, but it was so sexy because neither of us said anything beforehand. Anyway, now for some reason, he never does that anymore. He likes to call sex 'pokey-pokey,' which is not quite as erotic as turning off the lights in the bedroom and laying there naked, silently waiting for me. That was hot!"

Arlene and Sam need to rewind their sex life back to those early days when they had that nonverbal sexual tension. And it's not that hard to do. We suggested to Arlene that she should start things off one night by doing what Sam used to do—just waiting in bed silently with the lights off and seeing what happens. The results were even better than she had anticipated:

"Oh my God! It was the best thing I've ever done! I don't know why I didn't think of it myself. One night I did exactly what Sam used to do. I unexpectedly turned off the lights in the bedroom and just lay there naked. I was so afraid! I thought he might come in and say 'What the hell is going on?' but he knew instantly that I was lying there waiting for him, and I think it turned him on like he's never been turned on before. We made love like a couple of eighteen-year-olds! Then, the next night, he turned off the lights in the bedroom and waited for me. But this time, he hung a sexy negligee that he must have bought that day on the door. I thought that was so cool. Instead of saying something like 'Look what I bought for you,' he hung it on the door, which meant he wanted me to put it on. It was so erotic. My fantasies were all over the place that night. It was beyond hot!"

What happened with Sam and Arlene shows what can happen once we let our imaginations take over in the bedroom. Silence truly can facilitate that. Fantasies don't necessarily mean that we are thinking of someone else and not our partner when we are bed, but they do mean that we are thinking of each other outside of our usual reality.

This is why using a lot of words can be detrimental to getting out of your daytime persona with your husband. Your everyday voice and way of speaking, no matter how pleasing and sweet, will only remind you both of your out-of-the-bedroom selves. It won't conjure up thoughts within either of your minds of the sexual animals in you that have absolutely nothing to do with the woman who was making lasagna earlier that evening or the man who was fixing the leaky faucet. Your bedroom is your place of sanctuary, sexuality, and fantasy with your partner. So remember to treat it that way.

If you practice this often, your sexual world and your relationship as a whole will become a brave new version of the world it was before. A world where things are continually fresh. Sex should be a place where you go physically and mentally to escape from your daily world—where you feel different than you do during the day. It all starts with really taking that time to look at one another and letting your mind, not your words, take over from there. The only kinds of conversations you should be having in the bedroom (apart from good ol' dirty talk) should be soul-sharing kinds of conversations. Step back from your everyday selves and allow *real* intimacy to take place with nonverbal communication. Take that time for yourselves. Enjoy the simple wonderfulness of being close. Feel the warmth of skin on skin. Listen to each other breathing. Let your partner's touch affect you. And of course, look into each other's eyes. The power of this simple thing is huge.

CONNECTING WITHOUT WORDS

1 Take the time every day to really look into your partner's eyes. Allow those moments to let yourselves feel that strong connection between you.

2 Don't verbalize every thought that crosses your mind during the day, and promise not to have endless chatter in the bedroom about the daily chores. Your bedroom is your sanctuary—treat it that way.

3 Every day practice a few minutes of silence with your partner, and communicate using touch—whether you are in bed or not. Tune out the world and tune in to each other.

4 Don't bring a list of "intimacy needs" to bed with you. Don't dictate to your partner about sex; lead with your body instead.

5 Look into each other's eyes sometimes during sex, and have the courage to go where that takes you.

Chapter Five

Talk Dirty... Be Dirty

"I love it when my husband looks into my eyes and simply says 'I can't wait to fuck you.'"

—LUCINDA, AGE 38

"Whispering sweet filth into the ear of my lover always does the trick. Yum!"

—DAPHNE, AGE 29

IN THE PREVIOUS CHAPTER, we talked about the importance of nonverbal communication. And in earlier chapters we discussed how detrimental it is to your sex life if you and your partner call each other "honey," or silly names like (and get ready because we are naming and shaming): *baby-cakes, sugar-muffin, spoon one, spoon two, sweetie-kins, the pookster, booboo-poopdoop, honey bunch, dorkus, fatty-rumpus, bunchie, monsty, munchie-kins, bunny, sweetchips, nester-fester, cuddle-puss, mc-sexy, mc-muffin poopen cakes* (oh my God, after

McDonald's no less?), *lamby, lil-wuffers, boo-bear, poochi-kins, skittle-poot, tweenie-head, baberpants, shart* (um, isn't that pooing and farting at the same time? Nice!), *skumpy-furr, tuna, kookoo-liscious, schnicker-doodle, heffa-lumpie, shmoober, snurple, wubbahubbikins, uggums, sugar-butt,* and many, many more. We know it's been really *fun* to make up all these childish, cute, bizarre names. And, we know how creative we all are at coming up with some new cute and totally original form of "word" that we can now start using for our significant other. So, yeah . . . congratulations on those new heights of creativity. But we really need to stop all that now. Call your pet silly made-up names, have an imaginary nonsexual friend you can nickname, get a pen pal and call him or her something stupid, but don't do it for your partner. Maybe you simply needed to see this silliness in black and white to see the error of your ways . . . and stop!

So, you should now be addressing each other by your given names. This is vital because it confirms to our partners, both verbally and subconsciously, that we are separate entities. But it doesn't necessarily mean you should only call each other by your full first names—that can sometimes get a little boring too. For instance, if you have a name like Katherine, there are plenty of nicknames: Kathy, Kath, Kate, Katie, Kat, and so on. This adds a bit of variety but still maintains the difference between the two of you. That said, those variations are simply names we can use in polite company.

Give It to Me, Baby

Another name that you can call each other that is not necessarily detrimental to your passionate selves is "baby." But be careful! *Baby* is a very sexy word when used correctly and sparingly, so use it only during those sexy moments so it doesn't lose its impact. It is all too easy to destroy and desexualize a word. For instance, if you are saying things like, "Hey baby, can you take out the trash?" or, "Oh baby, I'm going to the supermarket to buy some tampons, do you need anything?"—that is definitely not going to work. You have essentially turned your sexy "baby" into just another form of "honey," "sweetie," and "pookie." And again, if you couple the saying of "baby" with those whiney, baby voices . . . well, you know the drill by now.

Use "baby" when you're feeling sexual with each other and want to flirt a little throughout the day. When you've missed each other all day, for example, say something like this to your husband when he walks in the door and you kiss him sexily: "Baby, I've been waiting for this moment all day long." Or, when your husband sees you looking really amazing, he can say, "Wow, you're sexy, baby." Get it? "Baby" is good, but don't misuse it. All those pop, rock, and soul songs can't be wrong! Smokey Robinson said it best with his song "Ooh, Baby Baby."

And don't shorten it to "babe" either—that's just a slightly better version of "honey." That follows too closely along the lines of, "Hey, babe, the cat barfed again, can you come help me clean it up?" Sure, Sonny & Cher sang "I Got You Babe," and that was a great song. But look what happened to their relationship. Our guess is that "babe" wasn't really cutting it.

So, "baby" is okay, but tread carefully. If you feel that by using even the word *baby* you find yourselves slipping into the dreaded "honey" scenario, then do not use it at all. Best to stick to your names and variations of those. Or, you can start experimenting with some juicier Anglo-Saxon terms, which leads us to what we really want to discuss. This chapter is all about what you might say to one another when no one else is privy to that conversation. We are talking about talking dirty. Yep, real smutty, down-and-dirty talk.

But before you can start getting in the frame of mind to be verbally provocative with your partner, you've got to make sure you're not doing things that make that next step impossible. For starters, you can't keep running around in your fluffy bunny slippers and comfy flannel nightie anymore while calling him "punkin" in that squeaky voice! How is that going to be seen by him as hot? Dirty talk, not cutesy talk, is the way to go here. Okay, maybe you really don't want to give up those fluffy bunny slippers and that comfy flannel nightie. But, you need to ask yourself honestly, would you have worn that when you first got together? No? Well then, maybe a trip to the Goodwill is in order. And for you guys out there, if you are walking around the house with that same old pair of ragged underwear with certain "items" hanging out, and a T-shirt with stains from multiple meals—even if you say something super sexy to your woman, it's gonna fall flat if you're looking like that, isn't it? If your underwear are ready to disintegrate if you simply blew on them, it's time to buy some new ones. Come on! Have some self-respect.

So be aware of yourselves, make an effort, and be mindful of how you appear. Now we are not saying that to talk dirty you also need to wear sexy clothes all the time or go to the gym 24/7, but there are levels of self-respect that you don't want to fall below. Going out and spending a small fortune on buying the latest Agent Provocateur or Victoria's Secret lingerie is not going to work if you are still calling each other "honey bunny." Even if you are lying on the kitchen table in a sexy pose, wearing high heels, stockings, a G-string, and push-up bra, when you say in your most babyish voice, "Oh, honnneee . . . look what I have for you," it's just not going to work. At a moment like this, you need to have something provocative to say to your husband—something raunchy or something alluring, and definitely something adult.

As with any long-term relationship, you've both got to make some effort. You all know this, right? You've made the effort with the communication, the partnership, the organizing of your daily lives, your chores, and the caring for your children (if you have them). But why have you left out the effort with regards to your sex life and maintaining your passion for one another? It's a very important part of your relationship that needs some attention too. So don't ignore that side of yourselves.

You need to step back and try to visualize your significant other as the person you are in a new relationship with, because the way to keep your sex life exciting is to keep it fresh. And here's the great thing . . . when you gain back that passion for each other, what you are rewarded with is better health and well-being. Your skin is better. You are more fit. You feel, and probably look, younger. You have a stronger bond. Yep, you get all that from having more sex. And it feels good! It's kind of a no-brainer. So, embrace the lusty, animal, earthy side of yourselves and talk dirty. Talk dirty and be dirty. Now we know that talking dirty can sometimes be easier for guys . . . they do tend to be more "up for it" in that respect, generally. But we aren't simply suggesting this for just your man to be turned on—we are suggesting it because it will turn *you* on. It's great for both of you. And trust us, as a woman, it will make you feel sexier and more in touch with your animal side. There's a full gamut of ways you can get in touch with that side of yourselves, so read on. . . .

To Porn or Not to Porn—
That Is the Question

One place to get inspiration for this kind of dialogue is from porn films. For those of you out there who might find watching porn distasteful and derogatory to women, we completely understand. We agree that there are undoubtedly many unsavory types, and even more unsavory practices, in the porn world. That's definitely true. And we are by no means saying that you should watch porn if it goes against your moral code. But even for you most upstanding girls and guys out there, there may be some phrases and things that can be taken from that smutty world and brought into your relationship. Why? Because it's fun!

One couple we spoke to, Tom and Sarah, were heavily into the retro scene. They both dressed in vintage clothes and were very stylish. For them, modern porn was just plain ugly and too crass for their liking. But, they did discover that they enjoyed adult films from the twenties, thirties, and forties. (Yes, believe it or not, they were filming people having sex the minute they invented the movie camera!) This may resonate with many couples today, even if they aren't into the retro scene. For Tom and Sarah, and many other couples, they liked the idea of watching something forbidden sometimes in bed, but they didn't like the super-raunchy, sometimes downright gross, aspects of modern adult films. So instead, they found what suited their sexuality and their tastes. That's what is so great about exploring your sexuality with your partner—you can find out what your mutual turn-ons are and learn more about each other as a result . . . and have fun in the exploration!

Now, let's think back again to when you were first together with your partner, and how much you wanted each other. C'mon . . . you did! You lusted after one another like crazy. And you possibly said some pretty raunchy things to each other at the time, or at the very least thought them. When a relationship is still new, it's the excitement and the newness of a man's body, his touch, and his penis that gets you hot, right? And likewise, for the man, the thought of touching, and holding and being inside the woman he's hot for is pretty much constantly on his mind. You couldn't get enough of each other! Even for those of you who might recoil at the thought of dirty talk, have you ever tried it? Sometimes, as Eddie Murphy so brilliantly illustrated in one of his stand-up routines, "When you get into bed, would you rather have somebody say, 'Oh, make love to me,' or grab the back of your head and say, 'Fuck the shit out of me!'?"

Gettin' Primal

Let's be open and honest with ourselves here, and start getting in touch with our primal, animal side. We *are* animals after all. Just because we wear clothes, go to work, have bank accounts, and maybe even go to church, doesn't mean there isn't a more wild, animal side to us. And it's not a bad thing! What, you feel guilty? Or trashy? Or it feels too derogatory? You and your partner already love each other, right? The commitment is there. You are together. And what got you to that point of wanting to commit? Are you gonna tell us that it was only about you two calmly and rationally discussing the "choices you both wanted to make in life," and you both made an "informed decision" to get together? Come on! You wanted each other, and you wanted it bad. There was love and lots of passion there.

Now that we have started taking the time to look into each other's eyes, we have to get down and dirty. Yes, we have got to up the ante, get earthy, and embrace that lusty, inner self that was just under the surface when you first met. It *is* still there lurking underneath it all. You haven't killed it, we promise. You've just got to awaken that smutty, inner animal.

Whisper While You Work

Rebecca and Sean have been together for nearly fifteen years. They have three kids, and they still have sex . . . a lot! When we talked to Rebecca and asked how she keeps it so hot that they still lust after each other after all those years—and with kids and all— this is what she told us:

"I'll be at work at my desk, and sometimes around a quarter to five when things kinda start winding down for the day, Sean will call me. When I pick up the phone, the first thing he'll say is, 'Hey, baby, what color panties are you wearing right now?' His voice is all low and guttural and sexy, so people don't hear him at his work. And I'll start giggling, and say something like, 'Oh, just a little black G-string.' And he'll say, 'Mmm . . . nice. Are you wet? Because my cock is getting hard just thinking about your wet pussy.' Then I start sounding all embarrassed and whisper something like, 'Sean! I can't talk about that now. I'm still working!' And he'll say, 'Okay . . . I just wanted you to know that I'm picturing you bent over your desk right now with your skirt around your waist, and my cock sliding into you as I bite the back of your neck.' 'Okay, Sean,' I say, worried that my coworkers are gonna hear me. And then I whisper even quieter, 'but only if you turn me over and finish me off lying on my back.' He then pauses a second to moan quietly, and he says, 'Oh yeah . . . I know how to make you come, don't I, you hot little bitch.' At this point I'm shuddering with that electric jolt of excitement that goes right up through my center. I then take a breath, compose myself, and tell him that we'll have to continue that, um, 'conversation' after work. For the rest of the time that day, I'm counting the minutes to when I can see him, and find a way for us to have at each other. When we do get together after work, the sexual tension is so hot, we can't wait to fuck. We barely even take time to take our clothes off, it's so hot and heavy! I love that about our sex life. We can always go to that fantasy place in our relationship and talk dirty to one another. Talking dirty keeps it alive for us."

Now we know that this kind of talk may be a little shocking for some of you. We realize that Rebecca and Sean's story might read like something from the letter pages of *Hustler* magazine. But talking dirty doesn't necessarily have to be quite this pornographic. For Rebecca and Sean, they found that talking really graphically works for them. Even if they come home to their usual house full of kids and aren't able to have sex right then and there, the sexual frisson they created earlier keeps them excited. They continue on with a look, a touch, or a suggestion, known only to them, until they can go to bed. Do you see how nonverbal communication *and* talking dirty can go hand in hand? The key to Rebecca and Sean's success is they have found ways to work dirty talk into their daily lives. They keep it unpredictable and exciting, and for them, extremely smutty!

But every person and every couple is different. Everyone finds that there are different things that get them going. For those of you who might not like that level of smut, imagine a slightly different scenario. How turned on you would be, for instance, if your husband called you up at your office, and said these simple words in an intimate voice, "Hey, baby, what color panties are you wearing? I just need to know." How would that play with your mind? Don't you think that having your partner just say something simple like that would really set your mind racing? Exactly. This is what we mean by talking dirty. Talking dirty doesn't need to be done every second of every day, however. We still have our daily chores and regular things to attend to. Talking dirty doesn't necessarily have to be pornographic either. But, you've gotta get creative with it, and find things that work for you and your partner. Choose your moments. Catch your partner off guard. Be unpredictable.

There should be no regular routine when it comes to how and when you get each other hot. You have a routine for your workdays and when you pay the bills. You might always have dinner at the same time, in the same place, but routine should not play into sex. If you have a routine date night, and you always go to the same place and do the same things . . . well, stop! If there is nowhere else in your life that you are thinking and behaving creatively, then let this be that one area.

The All-Important Audible

We all like little surprises from our partners—something unexpected that shows their love. Whether it's a box of chocolates, a dozen roses, or new perfume—when our man surprises us it usually gives a nice lift to our day. It puts a smile on our face and warms our hearts. Well, it's the same in the bedroom, too. We all need little surprises here and there, and the following couple's experience is a prime example of this.

Leon and Keisha had been living together about six years and were generally very happy. Like so many couples, they got along fine, were very good friends, but they didn't have the hot sex they had in the first few years. Until one day when Leon introduced "the audible." Keisha explains:

"Leon and I were at a place in our relationship that all couples seem to get to after five years, especially one that started with major pent-up lust like ours did. Our tapering off seemed inevitable given the amount of pure energy we had in the beginning. The frequency dropped, the passion dropped, and I think our general need for sex just fell off the charts. We talked around and around about it. We read many self-help books that suggested making a list of "intimacy needs," etc., but nothing worked. I think we were just a little bored with each other, to tell you the truth. We both knew what each other's moves were, so to speak, and everything became very predictable.

"One day Leon was going to the store to get some ice cream, and he asked me what flavor I wanted. I said, 'I don't know, surprise me!' I think I saw his face twitch a little when I made that simple remark. Believe it or not, that simple remark gave him an idea that really reawakened our sex life.

"The next time we found ourselves naked in bed together—you know, doing the usual stuff—there were no surprises, no complaints, and no changes to the usual sequence. You know . . . yada, yada, and then we were done. But then, out of nowhere, he flipped me into a position I had never been in, said some pretty raunchy stuff, and took me in a way I had never experienced before. It was exciting as hell! I asked him later how he decided to take a chance and do something different. He said, 'I decided to call an audible. That's a term in football when the offense lines up with the defense on the field and decides on a new play at the spur of the moment because of the way the other team is lined up. Well, I decided to surprise you with an audible.'

"From that moment on, we both felt less inhibited and started to try different things every once in a while. We've played around with new positions, dirty talk, and even some sex toys. I definitely feel that we're much more excited by each other again."

As Leon and Keisha found, sometimes couples need to do something bold to break out of the rut they're in. So don't be afraid to call your own audible with your husband! You don't have to surprise him with something shocking, like a super-raunchy sex toy, if you're not comfortable. Start with a minor little surprise and go from there. Chances are he'll take the bait, and start giving you some audibles too.

The important thing with all of this is that you two are seeing each other as sexual beings, as the former passionate lovers you were way back when—with more spontaneity, more surprises, and definitely more dirty talk. Now he can call you "baby" or "hot bitch." And you can call him "my stud with the hard cock." What is said is purely up to you, of course. You both need to discuss what kind of talk turns you on and how smutty you want the talk to be. Each of us is different in that respect. If your partner starts talking really dirty to you and calling you something like his "hot pussy" and that makes you feel uncomfortable, then obviously that kind of talk isn't going to work for you. Maybe instead, he could talk about "how much I want to be inside you and feel you underneath me" or "I really want to taste you right now and feel your legs wrapped around me." Now, if this kind of talk gets you going, then you need to tell him to say things like that. Or, if pretending you and he are someone else does it for you, then do that. All of this is good. Dirty talk, role-playing . . . the whole thing. The sky's the limit on what fantasies you want to explore mentally, verbally, and physically together. Again, personal creativity will keep it exciting. Start with that nonverbal communication, and then find your words and the ways you want to say them, and *mean* it, with all the fullness of your primal, animal selves.

Some couples can have a problem with talking dirty simply because their likes and dislikes in this area weren't communicated well enough to each other. The last thing you want to do is be saying the wrong things to each other thinking you are getting your partner hot, and instead, you have just thrown a big wet blanket over the whole thing! Unfortunately, that big wet blanket can turn into no sex at all. So, it's important to get this communication right. Both your and your partner's wants and needs are important, for giving and receiving. Neither of you should take a backseat on this. Up front and honest is the only way to be.

Be on the Same Page

Kara and Chase just got married recently. Both were married before and are now in their early thirties. Chase and his ex-wife had spilt up over their differences in what they considered to be dirty talk. And, although he and Kara are very happy, Chase's first marriage could have possibly been saved had he and his wife communicated their likes and dislikes when it came to their language in bed. Kara explains what had happened in her new husband's first marriage:

"Chase and I just got married not too long ago, and recently he told me that his ex was 'all weird' about what she called dirty talk in bed. First of all, she hated it when Chase said anything even slightly raunchy. He told me she would get really upset and offended if he said something as simple as 'I love sucking on your tits,' or 'You've got such a great ass.' Now, I consider myself a fairly mature and worldly woman, and while I'm not always prone to using dirty talk outside the bedroom, I do actually like it when we are having sex. But with his ex, Chase was telling me that she would say things like 'You have a nice penis,' or 'Please put your mouth on my vagina' or even, 'I need some moistness on my labia.' This totally cracks me up! It's no wonder he said that sex with her was a complete turn-off for him, and I can totally understand why. I mean, the words *labia* and *vagina* sound so clinical, it's almost gross. Her 'dirty talk' completely turned him off. Who wants to hear stuff like that during sex? How is that hot? If I were a guy, what would I rather hear? Let's see . . . 'Can you insert your penis into my vagina' or 'Fuck my hot wet pussy'? It seems like kind of a no-brainer to me! Thankfully we both have no problem talking dirty in bed . . . and the sex is pretty damn great!"

For Chase and his ex-wife, clearly their dirty talk was not on the same page. Chase and his first wife's main problem was definitely their poor communication. And it probably extended beyond the bedroom as well. Experimentation is good when it comes to sexuality, but not if there are things that you or your partner are doing or saying that are making you feel uncomfortable. If all kinds of dirty talk make you feel uneasy, it may be something a little more deep-seated in your psyche that needs to be explored. Sex is all in the mind. And the mind has to conjure up sexy thoughts for the body to respond. Dirty talk helps facilitate this. We just need to make sure that it's the right kind of dirty talk for each of us.

Sex with the one you love should be fun, it should feel good, and yes, it should sometimes be dirty! Smut is not a bad thing. You and your partner are simply celebrating your bodies together. It's even biblical. The Song of Solomon in the Bible's Old Testament talks exactly about the ravenous love (and lust) Solomon and his bride felt for one another. They explored it and rejoiced in it. There was nothing wrong with it then. And there is nothing wrong with it now.

Horny Is Human

You may be doubting this, especially now that you and your partner have been together awhile and you've "been there, done that." Or maybe you just aren't feeling sexual because you've just had a baby. Or you are busy . . . or tired . . . or you are "older now," or all of the above. Also, if you were previously calling him "sweetie-kins" and he was calling you "mommie bear" you might be thinking, *How in the hell am I gonna feel dirty and sexy again?* or *What inner animal?*

Or you and your partner may be thinking, *But our relationship is great, and we just don't have time for sex anymore. Besides, we're not that sexual anyway.* Well, there is a dark side to that. Remember in the introduction, when we talked about what eventually becomes of a relationship with little or no sex? Celibacy or cheating. And usually after a time of celibacy in your relationship, the cheating comes soon thereafter. Yes, really. You might think that you are "just not horny any more," or that you are "past that stage in your relationship" and you "just don't need it anymore." Well, think again. We are all human. Part of our humanity is our sexuality.

One or both of you will more than likely meet someone sometime in your life who is going to get your sexual juices flowing again. It happens. In fact, it happens all the time. Why do you think the divorce rate is so high? People are in humdrum relationships where they aren't having any sex. Or, even when they are having sex, they are simply going through the motions in a boring, routine way. But all of a sudden, someone comes along, and all these thoughts and feelings come flooding back just like you're a teenager again. And we aren't talking about a trickling stream that you may be able to cover up. We are talking about raging rapids!

How difficult is it not to want to act on that? Judging from the divorce rates or even just the statistics of people cheating on their spouses, those feelings are so intoxicating that it is very, very difficult to ignore them.

Some of you may think that you can put your sexuality away in a little box because you just aren't feeling it anymore. But trust us, that box (no pun intended) will burst open one day when someone you meet triggers it. Your sexuality will always find a way to come out again, no matter how convinced you are that it's buried forever. Kind of like those bits of grass that you see sprouting between the cracks in the sidewalk. Your sexuality has an incredible will to live, and if you aren't letting it live in your own relationship, it will sprout up somewhere else.

Remember the story of Brian and Megan in our first chapter? They were the couple who were together for twenty years and were great friends, but Brian had cheated on Megan and had gotten a woman pregnant as a result. Brian and Megan both thought they were happy, even though they had put their sexuality away in a little box. However, Brian's indiscretion was a result of his sexuality breaking out of the box he thought was locked tight. Some of you are probably thinking, *Oh. . . I bet he got together with some beautiful, sexy young girl.* And that could be possible. Or, he could have gotten together with someone who wasn't as attractive as his long-term partner. Their relationship was already deeply in trouble (even though they didn't realize it) with the "honey" talk, the baby talk, and being seemingly comfortable as only best friends. But with Brian and the other woman, the looks didn't matter as much as the nonverbal communication that started to take place between them and the kind of words they used.

Brian told us privately that this was why he couldn't help himself. It was the words that turned him on, he told us. "She just started talking really dirty with me one night and I couldn't believe how turned on I was," he said. "She wasn't even particularly pretty or interesting to talk to, but once we started our little dirty rapport with each other, I just couldn't help myself." That is the important thing to look at here. Do you think the girl was saying to Brian, "Hey, hon, you wanna come over to my place after our business meeting and maybe have some sex?" Very doubtful. There was some serious flirtation and dirty talk going on. She made some very suggestive comments, such as, "Oh Brian, you make me so hot, I'd really like to suck your cock right now." He then reciprocated with yet more dirty talk, and his sexuality sprouted up like the grass between the cracks in the sidewalk. At that point he was probably so turned on he simply couldn't stop. This is how powerful sexuality is. Once talking dirty started to come into play, he was already at the point of no return. If this kind of flirtation and dirty talk were going on at home, and Brian and Megan were mentally turned on by each other, would this other woman be such a strong temptation to him that he would throw his relationship of twenty years away? We don't think so.

Your Own Secret Language

As we explored in the first chapter, it's your everyday sexual dialogue that keeps your relationship hot. This is what Brian and Megan were sadly lacking. Your sexual dialogue starts with calling each other by your names and using your adult voices when speaking to one another. It also encompasses all of the other ways in which we communicate with each other throughout the day, both verbally and nonverbally. Dirty talk is another one of those ways.

Rebecca and Sean—with their phone sex while at work—have a very explicit way of talking to each other when they want to turn each other on, but not every couple needs to be this raunchy. Couples need to have their own secret language, one that they both feel comfortable with. This is vital in *every* relationship. It's kind of like having your own frequency or wavelength with one another—your own sexual shorthand in a sense.

Let's Swing a Little? Hmm . . .

When couples have lost this connection and they don't have the tools to get it back, it can be extremely frustrating. It's similar to being in your car and looking for a lost radio station that you used to love—you keep turning the dial and turning the dial and all you get is static. Then what do you do? You either turn off the radio—in this case your sex life—or you look for another station, as in another lover. And we highly discourage taking other lovers. Whether they are lovers you take secretly or you decide to be swingers together, it doesn't matter—even if you *share* in the experience. Just because you know about it and participated in the extramarital relationship, you think it's okay? It's not. Even if you stay together, it weakens that bond between you and creates a giant chasm in your relationship. That bond is for the two of you and the two of you alone. Fantasy is always better than the fallout from the reality. Even if one or both of you were to approach the extramarital relationship as "just a little fun on the side," we cannot stress enough how much that "little bit of fun" can deeply damage you as a couple and as individuals. Not to mention the fallout from the extramarital affair— even if your spouse knows about it—and how it affects your children, extended family, and friends. So don't do it! Even though we are saying that being dirty and talking dirty is a good thing, it doesn't mean that you should just go hog wild with the whole community! Go crazy and be lusty as hell with your own partner, just don't transfer that lust to anyone else. Again, that is what fantasies are for. Go ahead . . . fantasize like crazy, just don't make it a reality.

This is why we cannot stress enough the importance of having a great sex life, that is, a great sex life with your partner! If those feelings are not there with your partner, you or your partner will find it with someone else. If this side of your humanity is unfulfilled, nature will find a way to fulfill it. A long-term relationship is one of the most important relationships in a lifetime. Don't risk it by letting go of your sexual selves. When you are not sexually together anymore, an important bond is severely weakened. Sex isn't just about lust and fucking. Not at all. It's about bonding. It's the glue that keeps the bond tight.

Remember Irma and Guy in the first chapter and their "sex weekend"? Even though they were very happily married, they had lost their sexual wavelength and they didn't know how to get it back. They ended up watching old movies in bed and eating pizza during that weekend alone, like a couple of old girlfriends. A lot of fun, yes, but not exactly sexy. When couples get into "honey" this and "sweetie" that, and make no attempt to start talking dirty—the chances of having sex are just about zero. If they don't get back their natural sexual selves, it will only be a matter of time before one or both of them find themselves in a situation similar to Brian and Megan's.

Word Power

It is truly amazing, the power of words, and how they play with our subconscious. Words can make us women drier than the Mojave Desert, and alternatively, words can make us as wet as the raging rapids of the Colorado River. How do we wake those sleeping lions within us? Many of you can go back to the beginning of your relationship and start to do the things that you used to do with each other: take showers together, give each other massages, or call each other up in the middle of the day and say something suggestive.

All these things need to be done genuinely. Don't just go through the motions. Trying to talk dirty while having sex on the hood of your car in your garage when the spirit doesn't move you is just going to feel stupid! And contrary to what the "experts" advise, forcing yourselves to have sex is not going to increase your desire to have more sex. In fact, quite the opposite. Feeling like you *must* have sex definitely makes it yet another chore in the weekly grind, like taking out the garbage or doing the dishes. You feel like you want to get it over with, rather than relishing and enjoying the experience. So, if you ain't feelin' it, don't go there yet. It's got to feel right and natural to you and not stupid or ridiculous. It is totally pointless if you fake it.

But what if it's been so many years, you don't even remember what got you both going back then? Or, what if what worked in the beginning of your relationship won't work now because it was so long ago? You're different people now and what got you both turned on when you were twenty-five might not turn you on when you're forty-five. What then?

The nonverbal communication we talked about in the previous chapter is where to start. It sets the scene and the mood, and then talking dirty or suggestively will come naturally as a result. Both of you need to let those feelings wash over you again. Think of sex as a beautiful escape to an earlier, carefree time in your life—not one of your chores, but something that takes you away from your chores. In the beginning, you didn't think about those mundane things when you first met your significant other, did you? Seeing each other and being together was your escape time from everyday life. When your sex life with your partner is a welcome escape from the everyday realities, your relationship will remain strong. And when the connection between you and your partner is passionate and secure, those outside encounters will lose their power to damage that bond between you. The Stanley Kubrick film *Eyes Wide Shut* tackles exactly this issue:

In one scene of the film, Nicole Kidman's character (Alice) reveals to Tom Cruise's character (Bill) how she lusted after a sailor she only briefly saw when they were on a family vacation together. She tells him that if the sailor had approached her, she would have risked everything she held dear with Bill—her marriage, her daughter, her home—to have sex with this stranger. This seemingly brief encounter was that powerful for her. It was obvious at that point that she was lusting after a fantasy because she and Bill had no fantasies together anymore, and their lives had gotten a little mundane. Alice probably wouldn't have had such a strong urge to be unfaithful if she and Bill still had a fulfilling sexual relationship together. Remember in the beginning of the film, she pees and wipes in front of him, too? Bill and Alice fell into the same scenario most of us do: doing *everything* in front of one another, calling each other "honey," not talking dirty to each other, not being turned on much anymore, and definitely not having enough sex together. That glue had gotten pretty damn old and brittle. When Alice confessed her secret, Bill's sense of security and trust with his wife was completely shattered. Shocked and confused by her admission, he wandered the night debating whether to be unfaithful to her. Due to circumstances though, that didn't happen. But if things had been different? He probably would have cheated on her in revenge—maybe even more than once. Later in the film, all their truths come out. They talk in depth about what Bill went through that night and the sexual dreams and fantasies of Alice's, all the while renewing the communication between them. And it's important to note the last few lines spoken in the film:

Alice: I do love you, and you know there is something very important we need to do as soon as possible.
Bill: What's that?
Alice: Fuck.

Alice realized the importance that passionate "fucking" had in their relationship, and the necessity of renewing that bond. Again . . . and again . . . and again. Glue gets brittle. We need to keep the bond tight by continually adding new glue to our relationships.

Talking dirty and being dirty has many aspects: it's smutty, raunchy talk; it's mildly suggestive talk; it's about fantasizing together; it's a look, a touch, or a gesture; it's a secret language between you and your partner. The important thing is that it all helps to rekindle that sexual side of yourselves that should never be lost. Fucking is important. Fucking is deep. Fucking is fun. Fucking is all these things. And in your relationship, fucking, and sex in general, is absolutely necessary.

GETTIN' DOWN-N-DIRTY

1   Use words with your partner that make you feel sexy and maybe even a little smutty. Say what you feel and have fun with it!

2   Get creative and don't be afraid to be unpredictable. Call an audible every once in a while. Don't let routine take over your sex life.

3   Get in touch with your primal instincts and embrace your animal side. It's an important part of your humanity, so don't deny that part of yourself.

4   Set the mood with nonverbal communication, and let the words and feelings come naturally. If you don't feel it . . . don't say it, and don't do it. Remember that sex is an escape from your daily lives, not just another chore.

5   Rejoice in the love and lust you have for one another. Fucking is the glue that keeps you together.

Chapter Six

Argue More

"[We are] still engaged with each other, hot for each other. . . .
There hasn't been a moment when I have been bored."
—MARIA SHRIVER, SPEAKING ABOUT HER MARRIAGE TO ARNOLD
  SCHWARZENEGGER (*VANITY FAIR*, NOVEMBER 2004)

"You have to keep the fights clean and the sex dirty."
—KEVIN BACON
  (SCREEN ACTORS GUILD AWARDS, JANUARY 2009)

ARGUING IS ACTUALLY *GOOD* FOR your relationship. It may sound shocking, but it's true. When two individuals come together in a sexual relationship there is a clash of wills. This is a good and necessary thing. The friction created between two individuals coming together sparks the frisson that creates the desire within a relationship. And with that desire comes great sex. You don't necessarily need to have differences on subjects as strong as politics, the way

123

Maria Shriver and Arnold Schwarzenegger do, but you do need to have your own opinions and stick to them.

By arguing, we don't mean about serious stuff like the family budget or how to take care of the kids. We mean *playful* arguing. Yes, it's time to get feisty! Maybe you've never really tried this before, so please tread carefully. For instance, don't make fun of your husband's weight or job, but try poking fun at things like his taste in music or that stupid looking sweatshirt he likes to wear. But keep in mind, it needs to be clearly communicated what you both consider "fair game" when teasing or arguing with each other. So set some ground rules. If you say something that makes him feel low or bad about himself, then obviously that is a boundary not to go beyond. And likewise, if your partner says something that is very hurtful to you, you'll have to let him know. Don't forget to communicate those feelings—this is what good arguing is all about. Just remember that whether you are arguing or teasing each other, it's very, very important not to be disrespectful or deeply insulting. There is nothing worse than a couple putting each other down, whether in public amongst friends and acquaintances or in private. (Remember the "dead vessel" scenario in chapter 1?) This is the way feelings are hurt and resentment creeps in, so treat each other with care and respect—even when fighting. Like Kevin Bacon said, "You have to keep the fights clean. . . ."

Stand Your Ground

As women, we were often reared to be the compromiser or the mediator in the family. We probably learned this from the examples set by our mothers when we were growing up. But being the compromiser in the relationship often leads to the watering down of our own opinions and, as a result, our personality as well. We shouldn't let our opinions get swallowed up into the relationship. We need to hang on to those opinions and to those differences and fight for them. There will be times you may get exasperated with one another, but it will certainly keep you both fascinated and intrigued. Our partners can annoy us and make us crazy, but we want them even more because we want to tame their spirit! And here's the irony: even though we are each driven to tame the other's spirit, our spirits should never be tamed—because once we get what we think we want and conquer our partner, we are no longer as interested in them. Without the intrigue or frustration that occurs when your partner has different opinions from you, the necessary "frisson" is less likely to happen. We have all met couples who seem to be mirror images of one another. Most people view this as a good thing, but it is not necessarily so. If a couple agree on everything and have the same tastes and personality as each other, what excitement can occur? In these situations they get along just fine and are probably spooning regularly. But hot sex? Doubtful.

Jenny and Ben are a perfect example of one partner conquering the other and then losing interest. Married for five years, Jenny and Ben had much in common. They were both from the Midwest and had come to Los Angeles to pursue careers as musicians. Anyone who met them thought they were the most perfect couple in the world. They dressed alike—usually in black leather—and they agreed with each other on just about everything. They were both politically conservative, and they both loved eighties pop music, Chinese restaurants, rocker clothes, and old black-and white-movies. They were a very unusual couple who were so happy that they had found each other that they spent all their free time together. But what happened after a few years? Ben cheated on Jenny with—ironically enough—a woman who disagreed with his politics and who hates old movies! Ben explains:

"It was more my fault than Jenny's for cheating, of course, but I was just so bored after a while because she agreed with everything I said and kind of worshiped all of my opinions. In the beginning of the relationship we had a lot in common, but we did have differences of opinions on things like politics and movies. When we met, she wasn't as conservative as me on certain issues, but over time she started to agree with me on even my most conservative opinions. Also, when we met she liked modern comedies and didn't really appreciate old films like I did, and I used to make fun of her for that. I couldn't believe she liked to watch Meg Ryan instead of Carole Lombard! I was a bit of an ogre, I must admit. I kind of insisted that she agree with me on everything, and eventually she did . . . and that's when our sex life went downhill, unfortunately. Looking back on it, I kinda missed seeing her laughing while watching her silly Meg Ryan comedies."

As the breakup of Jenny and Ben's relationship demonstrates, when couples agree on every single thing, boredom usually sets in. When a man feels you are a complicated human being that he will never really fully understand or conquer completely, it keeps him on his toes and perpetually interested. Remember, he chose you because you were different from him, with different opinions and tastes. Men typically are aggressive conquerors by nature, but once they have conquered your spirit, they become bored and may move on to another conquest. Your spirit is something that should never be conquered, by your husband or anyone for that matter. He should not be able to predict your opinions on every issue. This leads to boredom, and boredom leads to little or no sex.

Playful Banter

Nothing gets those sexual fires going like a good playful argument. You need that kind of banter to keep your sex life alive. If you don't do this already, try starting now. For initial inspiration, start by watching *I Love Lucy* reruns, *The Thin Man* series with William Powell and Myrna Loy, any Spencer Tracy/Katharine Hepburn movie, and even episodes of *Cheers*. In the early episodes of the series featuring Ted Danson and Shelley Long, the characters Sam and Diane would often have heated arguments during their turbulent on/off relationship. In one particular episode they give a classic demonstration of the sexual tension that often occurs when couples quarrel. After an increasingly heated but playful exchange, the argument climaxes with the following:

> **Diane:** You disgust me. I hate you.
> **Sam:** Are you as turned on as I am?
> **Diane:** More!

The dialogue is followed by a passionate and lengthy kiss.

If you develop a good playful banter with each other, this will keep your sexual friction going well into your eighties, much easier than keeping a perfect figure and cheaper than buying lots of expensive clothes. Isn't this great news? All that working out at the gym or spending money on expensive clothes won't work as well at keeping you both interested as some simple new verbal skills in your daily life will. Playful arguing often leads to playful flirting, which usually leads to great sex.

Playful arguing shows your partner that you're up for a little verbal and mental challenge . . . and guys love a challenge! Sex is mostly in the mind, and when you show your mate that you have a provocative point of view, their interest perks up and the sexual fires between you begin to ignite. One thing to remember is that you should always argue or tease your partner with a smile on your face, so check yourself. If you're not smiling, you're not practicing playful arguing.

We need to think of playful arguing as yet another way of reaffirming your sense of self, both to him and to you. It shows your personality, your strength of opinions, and your fun and feisty character. And let's face it, this is what attracted him to you in the first place! By continuing to show you are different from him, you inadvertently continue to keep him interested in you. This is a more natural way of maintaining the excitement between you, rather than the more overt way of flirting, which often means you are trying too hard to please him and turn him on. Attraction and desire should be effortless. Be yourself, and he will come to you. Likewise, if he is doing the same, that keeps *you* interested as well.

You Annoy Me . . . but I Like You!

Remember back in grade school, when the guy you had a crush on was probably the guy who annoyed you too? Well, it's not that different when you're an adult. Adults can sometimes make the mistake in thinking that total agreement on every issue leads to greater compatibility. We acknowledge that it can be difficult to keep your own point of view in a relationship because we are naturally influenced by our partners and can sometimes adapt our views to theirs and vice versa. Granted, this is natural in some aspects of our lives, but you can carry it too far. When two people are interchangeable when it comes to viewpoints, it can be deadly for sex and the relationship in general.

Jared and Sally are a couple in their midfifties who have been together three years, yet they still live in separate homes. They are both realtors, working in the same office where they met. Sally admits that when she was first introduced to Jared, she didn't even like him:

"Jared came to our office about a year after I started, and he was very loud and made his presence known every time he was there. I even complained to my manager about him. But funnily enough, even though he annoyed me, there was something about his overly confident behavior that also attracted me sexually.

"We have a lot in common businesswise, which is a great thing to share, but in a lot of other areas we are very different. He hates the kind of restaurants that I like and my taste in music, and he's always trying to influence me in one way or another, but he never succeeds. I guess that's one of the great things about being a bit older—you know who you are, you know your beliefs and tastes, and you generally stick to them, much to the annoyance of a mate."

Jared explains his view on arguing and their sex life:

"In my first relationship, I was married for fifteen years, and she always thought that whatever I said was great, whether it was where to eat or what movie to go see. I was a record producer at that time, and she worshiped my taste in music, and all of my friends were her friends as well. And after awhile, we didn't have sex anymore, and I think it was because we never had any good banter going on between us—nothing to spark the sexual tension. I was pretty overbearing back then. I told her when we met, for instance, that I thought her musical tastes were uncool and, after a while, she finally agreed with me and started appreciating what I listened to. With Sally, it's totally different. Sometimes I can't believe her taste in things! One of the things she said when I first met her was, 'Well, everyone knows the Sex Pistols are the greatest rock band in history, and if you don't know that you know nothing about music.' She said that to *me*, and I'm a former musician and record producer. And she actually believes it! She thinks they were better than The Beatles! Everything, from her taste in food, her taste in music, and her taste in films, are things I'll never understand. She always sticks to her guns and tells me I'm just wrong, which irks me to no end. But our arguing is very playful when it happens, and I guess that's why we have such a great relationship. She's a feisty woman, that's for sure, and even though I may not agree with some of the things she says, it's always fun to listen to her! I still adore her."

Even in the very beginning of an encounter, it's extremely important to stand your ground and not be afraid to express yourself—

not only just to attract a mate, but to show your personality to the world. This may be difficult at times because we really want the man to like us, especially if we have just met him. Many of us find it hard expressing a different opinion because we fear running the risk of being rejected. But often, just the opposite happens. Men are generally intrigued when they meet a woman who has something provocative and interesting to say.

Julie, a twenty-three-year-old single woman living in Manhattan, has this to say on the subject:

"Many times I've been out with my girlfriends and we've ended up flirting with men at bars. They seem to take notice of me—not because I'm the prettiest woman in the group, but because I've challenged their opinions on something.

"Recently my two girlfriends and I were downtown at a very posh hotel bar after being at a daylong Microsoft convention. There were men and women from all over the world who came to hear Bill Gates speak and to talk about the company's new software products. After the conference we went to the hotel bar to relax and have a few cocktails. A cute, young Danish guy soon joined our table, and the conversation turned toward comparing Europeans to Americans and our supposed ignorance of geography. I remember he said something like, 'Most Americans don't even know where Denmark is on the map, or even that it's a part of Europe.' My two girlfriends immediately agreed with him and said, 'Yes, we Americans have no idea where other countries are located . . . we can be so provincial.' So I butted in and said, with a smile, 'Well, maybe that's because no one really needs to know where Denmark is!'

My friends looked at me as if I were the rudest person in the world and didn't understand how I could insult such a handsome young guy. I then went to bar and started chatting with some other colleagues I knew. Well, guess what happened? The Danish guy came over to the bar a little later and said he'd love to see New York with me and wondered if I was free the next day!"

What does this tell you? That you should always have your own opinions and use them to flirt a little. Being flirty and feisty is a good thing! Arguing more doesn't mean you become some argumentative bitch. That's a sure sex killer! What it does mean is that you need to hold on to your opinions, but you have to express them, as much as possible, in a humorous, charming manner. It's not easy though. As we've said already, we were raised to always accommodate a partner. We women are supposed to be the ones who make everything okay in the relationship. However, that makes for a very uneventful home life, and an uneventful sex life, too.

Dominic and Carrie met on an Internet dating site and have now been living together in Colorado for seven years. Dominic, thirty-nine, works as a civil engineer and Carrie, forty-two, is a teacher. Dominic says:

"There are certain things about Carrie that drive me crazy! I don't understand why she doesn't agree with me about things that seem so obvious. Her opinions are usually so extreme—she either loves something or she absolutely loathes it, and there's no middle ground at all. She's so obstinate it really annoys me, but she also turns me on at the same time!

I suppose I admire her passionate nature even though I don't usually agree with her. I know it's maybe weird to feel this way, but I've talked to other guy friends of mine and they feel the same. I mean, who wants a lapdog around that agrees with everything I say?"

Don't Put Him on a Pedestal

At the other extreme from Dominic and Carrie, we have the married man our friend Cynthia met at a bar. Cynthia is a very pretty fifty-two-year-old woman who works as a casting director in Hollywood. She has been single for the last five years, ever since her movie producer husband passed away. Recently, Cynthia was at a very exclusive restaurant in Los Angeles, waiting at the bar for a girlfriend to arrive, and she ended up talking to an attractive fortysomething movie executive about relationships. The movie executive said he had the perfect wife because she loved him unconditionally and she worshiped him completely. He explained to Cynthia, "I don't know if you know what it's like to have someone look up to you and absolutely adore you. I don't think I could ever give that up. She really, really loves me, and she only wants me to be happy."

His wife was home caring for their newborn. So Cynthia then asked him why he was flirting with her at the bar if he had this perfect relationship. He told her that even though he could never give up his wife, he didn't feel the same sexually about her anymore. He further explained how his wife's adoration and constant acquiescence had a detrimental effect on their sex life: "She worships me so much, and she practically hangs onto every word I say. Her whole life revolves around me. I'm everything to her. She always agrees with me, too, and I guess because of that, I'm kind of bored by her. It's almost impossible to conjure up the desire to want to have sex with her—even though I do still love her."

After this revelation he then suggested Cynthia spend a couple of days drinking vintage champagne with him in a suite at the Beverly Hills Hotel. Cynthia smiled and said, "I'm flattered, but I think you should really go home and tell your wife what you just told me. I'm sure your wife has a strong personality, you just need to help her uncover it." The movie executive was disappointed, but he gave her a peck on the cheek, picked up his martini, and politely excused himself so he could go on looking for another woman that night who might be more tempted by champagne and room service than Cynthia was.

Learn to Dance

Sexual chemistry between couples is like a dance, constantly moving and changing. The basics, however, stay the same. Sometimes you lead the dance, and sometimes your partner does. But when one dance partner does all the following and doesn't come up with any steps on her or his own, what happens then? A boring dance, and at least one very bored dancing partner.

Typically, men want to lead a discussion and to dominate it, whether it be with their partner or with a group of people. They probably learned this behavior from their fathers, just as we learned the opposite—to be compliant—from our mothers. Ever notice at a party how the men usually gather together to talk and the women usually do the same? Is it because the women want to talk about cooking or children and the men want to talk about sports? Sometimes, yes. But often this happens because men have learned the art of arguing from their fathers, and many women haven't. They like to talk to other men who can challenge their opinions on politics, art, religion, and more, and give them a good "run for their money" so to speak. We need to learn something here from men. We need to learn to be a little less compliant and a little more challenging in our daily lives, although in a playful and polite way. We gained so much from the women's liberation movement. Let's embrace some of those advantages: be politically and socially aware, have our own opinions . . . and yes, be willing to stand our ground and argue our points! This is just another area where we can show our individuality and keep our relationship healthy and interesting.

When we think of women like Lucille Ball or Katharine Hepburn, we think of two strong female characters who stood up to their men with spirit and wit. Try to inject a little of their attitude into your relationship with your husband, as our friend Susan learned to do in her second marriage. Susan and Tim have been together for ten years and still enjoy a great sex life. It's the second marriage for both of them, and they enjoy a playful banter with each other that Susan says was missing with her first husband:

"In my first marriage, I was much more serious and more of a wallflower. I know I probably got that from my mother. My father was a very domineering man who didn't like anyone to have a difference of opinion. He thought he was right on everything—from politics to how to open a can of tuna—and we weren't allowed to argue with him. My mother was never able to express herself at home and neither was I. So when I got married at twenty-two, I hadn't really formed my own personality yet. Consequently I just adopted most of the opinions and traits of my husband. All of his friends were my friends and all of my opinions were his as well. I remember every Friday night we would go out to eat, and I would say something like, 'Let's go wherever you want to go.' Even when my husband would beg me to choose where to eat, I would say something like, 'I really don't care, whatever you like, honey.' I was the 'whatever you like, honey' and 'whatever you say, honey' kind of wife. With hindsight, it was no surprise that he ended up being bored out of his mind with me, which led to him moving in with a girl he was having an affair with. I think in the beginning he found me very pretty and very sweet. But pretty and sweet only lasts so long before you want something deeper and more challenging."

After this first marriage dissolved, Susan went into therapy for five years and finally discovered her true self, which had never really come out in her life until then. She dated different men and got to know different kinds of people, both male and female, and gradually she discovered she did have some strong opinions after all. Susan discovered that she was passionately against animal cruelty, for example, so she started to volunteer at the local pet shelter. This is where she met and fell in love with Tim, the resident veterinarian. Tim recalls:

"When Susan told me she was the 'whatever you like, honey' wife to her first husband, I couldn't believe it! The thing I liked about her right away was the fact that she had such definite opinions on everything—from animals to where she liked to vacation to what kind of food she liked. Also, she had such a great sense of humor. One of the first things I remember is that she used to make fun of me because I liked to wear white loafers back then. She used to call me Pat, as in Pat Boone—that singer from the sixties who always wore white shoes—instead of calling me Tim. At first I thought, 'How rude,' but then I started to become interested in her. She's spunky and funny, and I like that."

Susan added:

"We tease each other constantly, which I never did in my first marriage because I guess I was emulating my mother back then. Tim and I constantly differ on a variety of topics, but we don't take it too seriously, because obviously we have enough in common that the relationship works. But I think the key is that we have enough *not* in common, and that's how the relationship works, too. I remember once he told me that he always wants to have sex with me because he said he's always 'a little agitated with me' about something. Weird, I know, but it works."

Much like Susan did in her first marriage, many women adopt the daily activities of their spouses—for instance, watching *Monday Night Football* or their favorite cop show. We need to ask ourselves: Do we really want to spend our free time watching endless sports and/or his choice of TV shows? Remember your time is your life—be careful how you spend it. Years of doing activities that you really wouldn't do on your own can go by without you even realizing it. By doing this, you are giving up your autonomy and your differentness from him. By not standing up for your own tastes and choices, you are becoming more of an appendage to him. Resentment will build up on your part toward him as well. Even if you think you are making him happy by going along with his requests, in the long term it will be bad for both of you. It will make him complacent about the relationship, and he could take you for granted. And you will both get bored. Fight for your likes and dislikes! Be unpredictable. Keep him on his toes.

Not the Hot Rod She Was Looking For

Jessica and Judd lived together for six years. They met at an insurance agency Christmas party and clicked right away. She found him easy to talk to, and he seemed like a free spirit, just like herself. He definitely wasn't the normal office-type guy, like most of the other men around her. One of his weekend passions was vintage cars, and, at first, she was very impressed that he had a pristine 1958 Corvette convertible. She explains:

"I always loved riding in his car on the weekends, with my hair blowing in the wind. It was so much fun, and I must admit I loved the attention. Everyone would stare at us and smile. I know it's so cliché, but it is pretty cool having a boyfriend with an unusual car. All the other guys at work drove really boring cars like Camrys and Accords, but Judd was different, and I guess that was one of the things that attracted me to him in the beginning. Unfortunately, he liked to spend almost every weekend going to vintage car shows or those specialist automotive shops. At first, when he wanted me to go to these places with him, I didn't mind because the relationship was new and I suppose it was something a bit different for me.

"But after a few months he got more and more into the car scene, and I started to really hate it. He always wanted me to dress up cute for him during the shows so all the guys would look at me standing beside the car. I felt like an additional 'car trophy,' which I didn't like. When I tried to suggest not going, he got all whiny and pouty, and guilt-tripped me into going. It became such a chore, and I really started to resent him for that. I work all week in a pretty boring job as a claims adjuster, and I started to hate that my weekends were filled with everything having to do with the stupid car!

"When we finally broke up, I realized how much resentment had built up and how that damaged our relationship to the point of no return. Looking back on it, I should've fought for my position more. But I guess I was hesitant to argue with him about it, so I just gave in and pretty much gave up. Now I know that if I had fought more for myself, I could've possibly saved our relationship. In the future, I'm not going to be so afraid to fight for how I want to spend my time. I mean, we all have to compromise a little, but there's a limit to how much."

The irony here, as illustrated with Jessica and Judd, is that although you may think that always going along with your partner's wishes to please him is going to help the relationship, the opposite is often true. Relationships need friction and arguing to survive, as strange as that may sound. Arguing means you are being honest with your partner and honest with yourself. And we've all heard the old adage *Honesty is the best policy*. It is.

So, arguing more doesn't mean you become a pedantic, argumentative person for the sake of it. It means you are a witty, playful, centered woman who is not afraid to express a contrary opinion. Your views are important, and so is your willingness to be honest and forthright with your partner. Just because you listen to him and consider his ideas, tastes, and opinions doesn't mean you forget your own. A great relationship is one in which both partners freely express themselves without fear. Remember, he picked you because you were different from him, because you challenged him, and because you intrigued him. Don't let that slip away.

FIGHT 'N' FLIRT

1   Don't dilute your personality just because you are in a relationship. Keep it strong and feisty.

2   Always argue with a wink and a smile. Keep it fun and humorous, taking care not to "punch below the belt" with your jibes.

3   If you catch yourself saying, "Whatever you like, honey" too often, stop right there, and speak your mind! (Need we mention the "honey" thing again?)

4   Every so often, reexamine your tastes and opinions. Are they really yours? Or are they his?

5   Don't be afraid to drive your partner a little crazy. Being annoying can actually turn him on!

Chapter Seven

Stay Separate to Stay Together

Husbands and wives should have separate interests, cultivate different sets of friends and not impose on the other. . . . [Joanne and I] are very, very different people and yet somehow we fed off those varied differences and instead of separating us, it has made the whole bond a lot stronger."

—PAUL NEWMAN, ON HIS MARRIAGE TO JOANNE WOODWARD
  (*PAUL NEWMAN* BY CHARLES HAMBLETT)

In any relationship, after the first year is over, you can't help but want your own space. Having two houses means that we can get out of each other's hair. I'm very happy."

—HELENA BONHAM CARTER (*GUARDIAN*, NOVEMBER 2006)

NOW, WE ARE SURE THAT SOME OF YOU read this chapter heading "Stay Separate to Stay Together" and thought, *What? I don't want to separate; I want to get closer and have more sex. That's why I'm reading this book!* Well yes, that is the point of our book—to get you and your partner to have more sex and to strengthen the bond between you. But unlike so many other books, we don't want to treat the symptoms, we want to get to the causes. And one of the causes of a declining sex life is the boundaries between two people become too blurred. What we have to realize is that a healthy relationship is not about becoming so close that you become fused into one entity. We must not let our individuality get sucked into the powerful quicksand of the relationship and swallow up our sex life along with it.

So, a little separation is a good thing. It allows your partner to see you outside the roles of wife, mother, and friend—the roles that you are in all day long. He is able to see you not as just a part of the family unit, but as an independent woman. No matter how scary that may seem to both of you at first, having a part of your life totally separate from the family is a good and necessary thing. Now by separation, we don't necessarily mean separate vacations, separate lives, or separate homes—although separate homes seem to work quite well for Helena Bonham Carter and Tim Burton. What we do mean, however, is that it is hugely important for you to maintain a separate identity from your partner. Your partner can never and should never know you completely, so a little mystery is definitely in order here. We are attracted to those who seem elusive, who we cannot totally control or understand. That's the nature of sexuality. Conversely, we are not attracted to someone who constantly clings to us, who we can totally control and understand. That's the nature of sexuality, too.

This may sound harsh, but your husband does not always want to have sex with you when you are in the role of wife and mother.

That doesn't mean he doesn't love you and find you sexy. What it does mean is that the roles of wife and mother are not *necessarily* sexy. And comparatively, the roles of husband and father aren't always sexy either. And we can bet that a lot of men out there don't want to have sex with the wife who was vacuuming the house all day, or the mother who made peanut butter and jelly sandwiches for the kids in the morning and who was changing dirty diapers an hour before bedtime. Even if that woman is his wife. He wants to have sex with the woman outside of that role. Likewise, you need to view your man not solely as the husband or father, but as the multifaceted and enigmatic man that he is. When you met each other, you obviously weren't a role to him. You were just you: independent, funny, mysterious, and interesting. All of the things you still are. You need to encourage that part of you to flourish again. And the only way to do that is to have a little separation from your partner to allow your true self to once again rise to the surface.

One of the reasons a partner will sometimes cheat is to have sex with someone they can look upon as a sexual creature and not as an appendage of themselves. People who go from relationship to relationship tend to do this because they want to have sex with someone before they become a role to them. But once the newness wears off, these people usually fall back into their respective relationship roles, and the cycle of cheating starts all over again. This is why the constant search for a new partner is so futile.

Couples that stay together in a long-term relationship tend to be happier and more content with their lives as a whole than people who flit from relationship to relationship or fling to fling. A long-term relationship is a constant in people's lives that gives them a solid grounding and makes life even more meaningful.

Throughout the lifetime of our relationships, we need to continually keep our own opinions and interests and make sure we are not losing our identity to keep the relationship going. Arguing, which we talked about earlier, is a necessary catalyst for the separateness to happen. But now that we've stood up for our opinions—and yes, even fought for them—how are we going to continue to back them up? The way we do that is to step away from our partners a little and learn to center ourselves again. Stepping away from your partner and getting back some of the autonomy that you had in the beginning is vital if your sexual relationship, and your relationship as a whole, is going to last.

As women, we unfortunately tend to become more enveloped in the relationship than is healthy and we can then lose our sense of identity in the process. When two people get together and become one in everything, from opinions to calling each other "honey," there is no sexual connection to be made because you are just too damn alike! How can you build a sexual bond between two people when you aren't two separate people anymore? As individuals, we need to have our own friends, tastes, and style. You already know all of your likes and dislikes, but if you and your partner are so close that his likes and dislikes are exactly the same as yours, then where is the interest? Of course you can have many things in common, that's quite normal. But if your relationship is so insular that you find yourselves building a wall around it to keep the rest of the world out, you are definitely too close and you aren't bringing anything new to the table. So check yourselves.

And how does this translate to excitement in the bedroom? It doesn't. Frankly, the more entwined you and your partner become, the more sex just becomes boring mutual masturbation. And if it's not exciting anymore, why do it? The result usually leads to little or no sex, and, as we discussed earlier, that can be seriously damaging to a relationship.

Sex thrives on the frisson between two individuals and the excitement of physically and emotionally connecting with another person. How we communicate, how we conduct ourselves, and how we feel about ourselves in our own lives, before we go to bed, determines our desire for one another. We've all seen couples that are too close or too alike—in our own relationships and in the relationships of our friends and families. How many times have we heard couples referring to their partners as "my other half" or "my better half"? Contrary to conventional belief and (dare we say it again) the "honey brigade," this is not good. It's so commonplace that none of us even thinks about the connotation of what calling each other "my other half" actually means! However tempting it is to get super cozy with your partner, it is the tension and friction and fascination of being two separate people that keeps the fire alive. The trouble is, when you ignore this original separateness—you do become each other's "other half." And that is simply too boring for either of you! When you relate to each other as separate individuals rather than just "the other half," it's going to be a lot more exciting.

To illustrate further why it's not good to become too entwined, just ask yourself how boring it would be to have a conversation all day with yourself? The kind of conversations you have with yourself waiting in line at the DMV or in a doctor's office? You know, that boring inner dialogue that just passes time and which you'd rather ignore. Are we bored yet? Yep. But imagine if you've just met someone that you really liked and desired, and they have something completely new to say, wouldn't you be all ears? The way they speak, and the phrases and words they choose are different from yours. They are saying things that you don't normally hear, which can be exciting and intriguing. It's normal for a couple who have been together awhile to have similar ways of speaking and similar thought patterns. But if this continues unheeded, it will make the two of you actually start sounding like the same person. This is the true road to boredom. Instead, by having separate interests and friends, you continually bring new thoughts, ideas, and phrases into your relationship with your partner. This will keep the relationship interesting and constantly growing and evolving. It allows us to repeatedly see one another in a whole new light and makes our desire for each other stronger.

So what *can* a couple do to get that separateness back and rekindle the flames of passion? A start would be adding new interests to our lives other than our partner, our children, and our home life. And we aren't talking about taking up a casual interest in needlepoint! This kind of hobby, and others like it, are things you can do while you and hubby are watching TV, yet again. Night after night after night. Yep, that is pretty darn unexciting. What we are talking about, however, is doing things you are truly passionate about. Having interests and activities that can really have an effect on you—the core of you—and take you out of your normal home environment. And if you don't know what those are yet, then you seriously need to take some alone time for yourself and discover (without your partner's help) what really floats your boat.

As Virginia Woolf wrote so beautifully in her classic essay *A Room of One's Own*, every woman needs a place apart from her husband and family where she can explore her true self and be creative. A place, she writes, where there is "No need to be anybody but oneself." Prior to 1929 (when the essay was written), she laments that only women with money and privilege could have afforded this simple luxury. But nowadays however, most of us are fortunate to have homes and lives where we can easily indulge in some alone time—which is important for women *and* men alike. Although this essay was written over eighty years ago, its message still rings true: to really sparkle, discover our true selves, and unleash our creativity, we need some separation and space from our partners.

Now, it's true that couples get together in the first place because they have things in common. For instance, they like the same music, food, art, or outdoor activities. All of this is normal and great, because it means that the couple has things they like to do together. But after a few years of exploring all those things they both love, then what? This is when a little effort has to be made to bring something new into the relationship. This shouldn't be an effort that feels like hard work, either. Taking the time to explore your life and yourself more fully should be fun and exciting!

Wanna Eat in Front of the TV Again, Honey?

Andrea and Carl have been married for twenty-three years. Since their two sons have both left home to attend college, they are now alone again for the first time in many years. Instead of enjoying their new privacy and freedom, Andrea and Carl feel lost and bored without their kids there to occupy them. Andrea explains:

"When both of our kids moved out of the house, there was such a hole in our lives. The kids always had new things they were into, and new friends they'd meet and bring over, so I guess we lived our lives vicariously through them, which probably wasn't healthy for Carl, myself, and our relationship. I'd socialize with the other moms, and Carl would sometimes go to baseball games with the other fathers and the boys.

"When the kids left, so did all of our excitement. Each night we just sit on the couch and eat dinner while watching our usual TV programs, not really talking or even looking at each other. Then later after dinner, I'll curl up on the couch, and he'll sit on the lounger, and we just while away our nights watching TV and not really talking much. Then one of us gets up and goes to bed—usually me first—and then Carl will eventually follow about an hour later. By that time, I'll be asleep. So, sex is practically nonexistent. Thinking back, I can't even remember the last time we've had sex. When the boys were still living with us, however, we used to look forward to them going to camp or for a sleepover at a friend's house because we knew we could have the house to ourselves and have sex anywhere—even on the couch if we wanted to! We were just happier back then because the house was always full of laughter and activity. When the kids were in the house, we'd always have issues to discuss with them and each other. Whatever the boys were doing or planning that season, month, or week was always the topic of discussion and the center of our lives. But now there doesn't seem to be much there for us to discuss or explore. We are both bored. I can feel that we've grown tired of each other, but I don't know what to do about it. I'm really depressed lately, and I think Carl is, too. But we don't talk about it. We always felt that our relationship was so good, but now it feels embarrassing to admit we have problems."

Just like David and Nicole (the two nurses in our last chapter who liked to "veg out" in front of the TV), Andrea and Carl also fell into the all-too-common habit of TV addiction. It's a sad fact but many people use TV as an escape from dealing with or confronting their problems. Couples worldwide get into the practice of passively staring at the TV. Or they become so immersed in entertainment programs or other people's lives on reality TV, that they don't take the time to concentrate on their own lives, relationships, and of course, sex lives. It's all too easy to spend hours watching TV and not look at the issues in a relationship that aren't working. Andrea and Carl are a perfect example of a couple who are not bringing anything new to their relationship, and they unknowingly use TV as a crutch to take the easy way out. Once their kids left home, they realized how stagnant their own lives had become. But did they deal with it? No. They chose instead to bury the problem by watching TV, night after night. Consequently, their sex lives suffered, which in turn, threatened their entire marriage.

The cure for this downward spiral is to make more of an effort with your individual lives and explore life a little more. Wouldn't you rather have your own lives be more exciting so that you don't feel the need to be entertained by watching other people's lives and stories on TV? Why live your life vicariously through them? Make your own life interesting so you don't need to be entertained by someone or something else. This means opening up to finding new things you can get excited about, have a talent for, and really love. That excitement and passion will in turn be exciting for your partner, too. In essence, he gets to discover new and interesting things through you. With that, comes a renewed interest in you, and in having sex with you.

Ideally, you and he should be ever changing and evolving. And if you're not, then you are simply not living life as you should—either together or separately. As Woody Allen said in the film *Annie Hall*, "A relationship, I think, is like a shark. You know? It has to constantly move forward or it dies." Don't let television take all the excitement out of your life. Switch it off, and get out and do things!

However, once you've developed this newfound *joie de vivre* it can't be one-sided. You both need to search within yourselves to find what really thrills you, and bring that excitement back into your relationship. If you find these suggestions difficult to incorporate into your partnership, take some small steps first. Maybe you once belonged to a book club, a hiking group, a volunteer group. Great! Rejoin them. These are the kind of activities that will help you recapture your sense of self and bring new experiences into both of your lives.

The Art of Attraction

Rick and Mandy had been together nine years and unfortunately, as with so many other couples, boredom had definitely set in. Although they had no children, their jobs kept them busy and their social lives were pretty predictable, as Mandy recalls:

"Although we have a pretty wide circle of friends and went out two or three times a week, we always went as a couple. Going to see films, going out to dinner, to parties—

you name it—we were kind of inseparable. Of course, for the first few years you enjoy the fact that you're always together and kind of a team. But we were together so much that it got to the point that I no longer saw Rick as my lover, but more as a best friend or a brother. We were so close that sex became almost awkward, like I was doing it with a close relation. There were no surprises left for either of us. Luckily, a good friend of mine started going to an arts and crafts class in the evening, and because she was kind of nervous about going on her own, she wanted me to go with her. Rick didn't mind, so I went along.

"To my surprise, I had a blast! I guess there was this artistic side of me that had been dormant for years because I just couldn't get enough of those classes! Sometimes I'd go with my friend or some of the other people that I met in the class to local art exhibitions. I got really good at oil painting, and I think Rick was surprised at both how much I enjoyed it and how good I was at it. Also, I think he was finding a new sense of pride in his wife, which was cool.

"My ego got a further boost because one of the art teachers was very flirty with me. He wasn't my type, and I wasn't the slightest bit interested in him, but it felt great knowing another man besides Rick found me attractive. I felt really alive again and because Rick and I weren't seeing each other every moment of every day, we started to appreciate each other a lot more. And for a change, we actually started having a lot to say to each other. I mentioned to Rick that the art teacher was flirting with me, and he got kinda jealous but in a good way. Our sex got better and better! I think he was seeing me as a whole new woman again.

"Because Rick saw how being artistic had such an impact on me, he decided to try creative writing for himself. This was something that he had always wanted to get into, but for some reason he hadn't pursued it. He loves it now, and I think it's given him a new lease on life. In fact, he's even started working on his first novel, which we are both really excited about. Now both of us have so much to talk about and experience together, it's great!"

Rick and Mandy are a great example of how when one person broadens their horizons, his or her partner can be influenced in a positive way and follow suit. This is not only good for each person's own life fulfillment, but it's also wonderful for the relationship. Bringing new interests and experiences into a relationship is like a breath of fresh air in a stagnant room. You will feel young, invigorated, alive, and yes, even sexy!

Unfortunately, not all partners are as receptive to new experiences as Rick. Sometimes problems can occur when one partner tries separation and new activities and the other partner stays stagnant. Always keep in mind that you are not only seeking to enrich your own life but also the life of your partnership. We need to help and encourage each other to explore new things. Don't get so carried away with your new activities that you forget your partner's thoughts and feelings. Remember, this is supposed to be a positive experience for both of you, one that will give you a more exciting connection with your partner. Even if your partner seems unreceptive at first, try to lead him gently out of the rut you're both in. He will thank you later!

Go the Distance . . .
but Don't Run Away

Greg and Sophie are in their late forties and have been together for almost twenty years. Sophie works part-time as a legal assistant and Greg is a busy full-time attorney. Now that their two children—both girls—are in high school and have become much more independent, the couple finally have some free time for themselves. Unfortunately, because Sophie had always been so involved in her children's lives, she found herself at a loss about what to do with her free time. She enjoyed athletics in high school and did very well on the track team back then, so she decided to take up long-distance running to get back in shape. It soon became her daily passion:

"It started out as a hobby to get myself back in shape, but soon it became kind of an obsession and my whole focus in life. If I didn't run at least five miles a day I'd get really depressed. I was totally driven! Meanwhile, however, Greg was just getting lazier and lazier. He got heavier and became even more of a homebody. I was really disappointed because I'd hoped that by seeing me start running again, it would influence him to get off the couch and get fit with me. Unfortunately, it didn't quite work out that way. It seemed that only I was making an effort to improve myself, and he was becoming resentful of the time I spent away.

"Soon I was entering out-of-town competitions and spending more and more time away from home and Greg. I had hoped that in the second part of our lives Greg and I would have grown together and found new passions in life. But it was clear that I was the only one trying to do that. I started to resent him because he was seemingly so lazy and didn't want to do anything.

"That's about the time I met David, another runner, at one of my out-of-town events. We became good friends and talked on the phone a lot. There was a time there that I seriously considered having an affair with him and possibly leaving Greg. I mean, David was so fit and so energetic, and Greg was such a couch potato. I just didn't want to have sex with Greg much anymore, even though it seemed like he wanted me sexually more than before. Greg and I still loved each other so much though—we have our kids together and invested so much of our lives to each other—and I didn't want to lose all that.

"So instead of making such a tragic mistake, I decided to talk to Greg about all my building resentment toward him and my fears that we were growing so far apart it couldn't be mended. We really talked about everything and tried to make it work out between us. It was a tough time for both of us, but I think it was a necessary thing for us to go through. We realized that we both had to put some effort into our lives as individuals to make our lives together more interesting.

"Greg also made me realize that I was being too selfish because I wasn't keeping in mind that we were still a team. It was stupid of me to consider ending our relationship simply because Greg wasn't interested in long-distance running. At the same time though, Greg also realized that he needed to make an effort to find new activities and passions so that he could lead a fuller and healthier life.

"Recently, Greg started playing tennis with a few buddies. He's really excited about playing again, and starting to feel more confident about himself as a result. Now we both have new things in our lives we can share. I'm going to start playing tennis with him soon, and we also plan to go hiking together. It's finally feeling more right again between us, and we both feel like we have a new lease on life. And I feel like our sex life is finally getting back on track, because I've become more attracted to him again. I'm so thankful that it's working out because it would have been such a shame to walk away after all the years we've spent together."

Sophie defeated the purpose of separation by letting her new interest become an obsession—an obsession that almost destroyed her marriage. When your activities get to the point of excluding your partner from your daily life, this isn't the kind of separation that helps your relationship grow. Always remember that you two are a team. For teamwork to work well, each individual has to make an effort. The point is not to explore so much of yourself that you've "explored" yourself right out of the relationship!

It's not a bad thing when you do activities separately, whether it's you going out with your girlfriends or him going camping or sailing with his guy friends. It gives you another dimension to yourself that your partner hasn't experienced with you. And it gives you that little bit of mystery too. He doesn't know exactly what you did, and who you spoke with or maybe even flirted with! But what it does is confirm that you both are still thriving individuals, and yes, still attractive to others. This gives you and your partner confidence in yourselves and rebuilds some of the intrigue and mystery that you had in the beginning of your relationship.

Waiting for
Your Prince Charming

Some of you may be in a slightly different situation. After thinking about your own interests and passions, are you saying to yourself, "Wow, it's been so long I don't even know what those are! My personality has been so tied up in 'us' that I don't know where to begin finding my true self." Try thinking back to the beginning of your relationship and ask yourself if you truly were your own person back then. Or were you simply a meek individual waiting for a Prince Charming to fulfill all your needs and desires? When he came along, did you think, *Now my life is complete and my prayers have been answered. Now I finally feel like a whole person.* If you are that yearning, hopeful Cinderella looking for that Prince to complete you . . . well, you've got some work to do. We should know—we've been there too.

From bitter experience, we can tell you that this isn't an ideal or comfortable place to be, either in your head or in your heart. Here's the trouble with being that hopeless romantic: it usually is hopeless, and it can be painful, too, because you're always chasing a fantasy. This kind of romance is great for a day, a week, or even a month or two, but in a long-term relationship, it's just not based in reality. Making your partner the absolute center of your life is dangerous. It is dangerous to your own spirit, and ultimately, it is unfulfilling and leads to deep unhappiness. If your relationship is based around your partner being the center of your existence, you must change that situation. Clinging to your man and expecting him to fill a void in your life is simply not healthy. Even if you feel he is filling that void now, we promise you that feeling will not last.

Sex, like love, shouldn't be needy. You shouldn't need him to make you feel complete sexually or otherwise. Sex should be something you want to have, not need to have. And frankly, if the sex you are having is because you feel you need it, you are never going to be fulfilled or satiated—no matter how many orgasms you may or may not have! It also isn't going to change that deep feeling of yearning, no matter how long you hold him and cuddle him before and after sex. And ask yourself—do you really want sex? Or is the wanting coming from a place of desperation or emptiness within yourself? If you are depressed or filled with angst and yearning for him all the time, then there is something missing in you. This is not real love. It is obsession. *You* need to fill that void in your life, not him. He should be an addition to your life. He should be a compliment to you. But he doesn't complete you. He doesn't define who you are. You do.

But What Am I Supposed to Do?

Marie and Justin were high-school sweethearts, but like many childhood sweethearts, they broke up and went on to other relationships. During a chance meeting at a mutual friend's fortieth birthday party years later, sparks flew between them once again. Because Marie was in the middle of a separation with her current partner and Justin was already divorced, they started seeing each other again after all those years. Marie explains:

"When Justin and I first got together again, I gotta tell you, it was just magical. It was like all my prayers were answered. I had been in some really shitty relationships before that. Now that my marriage was nearly finished, I guess I looked to Justin as kind of my lifesaver and my way out. My husband was never there for me anymore, and it seemed like he didn't want to spend time with me. The more I wanted to be with him, the colder and colder he got. I was nearly at the end of my rope with that relationship.

"Anyway, when Justin and I first slept together again, it was the most intense sex of my life, and I'd never felt so close to anyone as I did with him. It was so incredible. I realized then that he was the one I was meant to be with forever. Unfortunately, I was living about four hours away from him—which was pretty frustrating and really inconvenient—so I quit my job and moved in with him. Neither of us had any kids or ties really, so it was pretty easy to make the move. He told me that he was fine with me not working, so I stayed home and just did the wifely things: cooked, washed and ironed clothes, cleaned the house, and all that stuff. I had a few hobbies I guess, like gardening, and I liked to go on the Internet now and then. But for the most part, I wasn't really doing very much. I loved being with him so much that all I really wanted to do was be with him and do whatever he wanted to do. No matter how much time we spent together, I never felt like it was enough.

"After a while though, he would say he wanted to go out with his buddy Jim or go fishing for a few days with his guy friends. I would be like, 'But what am I supposed to do while you're gone?' I know he does spend a lot of time with me, but when he's away, I really feel like my life is on hold until he comes back.

"Lately I have been trying to have sex with him even more—thinking that if I'm eager for sex all the time, he'll want to stay with me and not go out with his friends. But even when we are together, it's like I can't get close enough to him. No matter how many times we have sex, it's just never enough. And ironically, now he hardly ever wants to have sex at all. And for me, I guess sex isn't really enjoyable anymore. I'm just trying to use it to hold on to him. But I'm starting to feel like I'm losing him. I've been really depressed and crying a lot, and now he seems to make even more excuses not to be with me."

Marie is in a very painful place in her life. And the mistake she is making (and quite possibly made in her last marriage as well) is that she does not have enough going on in her own life. Marie's definition of a relationship is that both partners' lives should solely revolve around each other. For her, Justin is everything: her emotional center, entertainment, sole companion, and reason for living. Because Justin has other aspects to his life besides his relationship with Marie (his work, friends, and other activities, like fishing), he can never fulfill all of her needs and give her the amount of attention she so desperately desires.

The romantic notion of "happily ever after" does not work unless you are willing to find ways to enjoy your life without your partner with you all the time. When you are happy by yourself and with yourself, your partner is more intrigued and happy with you, too. He will also quite probably want to spend more time together, not less. Why? Because you are interesting and fascinating to him! Although it does seem more common for women to readily allow themselves to get "swallowed up" by their relationships, this does occasionally happen with men as well. Both sexes need to be aware of this issue. We understand how easy it is to fall into a scenario similar to Marie and Justin's. We must fight against it, though. It's work, we know. But it's work that must be done for you to be happy in your life—whether you are in a relationship or not.

So, take some time away from him and your daily routine. Go for spa or yoga weekends somewhere with a friend or even on your own. Get into nature, read more, explore life, go out with friends, have fun, and get creative. And do it for you! Don't be afraid to be idle for a while either. Sometimes we are so busy with our daily lives that we have forgotten some of life's simple pleasures, like taking a walk in a park, or watching a sunset. Virginia Woolf also wrote: "It is in our idleness, in our dreams, that the submerged truth sometimes come to the top." *A Room of One's Own* doesn't necessarily have to be a place that is far away from your partner either. You can still have your own space and both be in the same apartment, or the same house. Go ahead: read, write, draw, meditate—whatever you feel like exploring in your life—as long as it's something solely for you. Get to know *you* again.

As individuals, we are constantly evolving. This is normal and natural. The goal is to evolve separately—but together—with your mate. We know this sounds like a contradiction in terms, but it does work. You should both be growing and changing as individuals, and then regrouping and coming together to share of yourselves—your new passions, thoughts, and opinions. This is how the relationship stays fresh. And this is how the sex gets hot again. When you keep the relationship fresh in this way, your desire for sex will be continually renewed. You are intrigued by each other again. You are excited by each other again. And when your minds are revitalized, your bodies will soon follow. Staying separate *will* bring you together and keep you together.

SEPARATION IS GOOD

1   Explore yourself *outside* your role in the relationship. Relish the many aspects of your individual passions and creativity.

2   Remember to allow yourself the space for "a room of your own" —a place where you can be yourself, without your partner's influence.

3   Always try to bring something new to the table in your relationship— new friends, ideas, activities. This will keep your relationship fresh, help you to maintain some mystery, and revive that sexual tension between you.

4   Don't be so focused on your new activities that you forget you are part of a team. Passion doesn't mean obsession. Don't exclude your partner from your life.

5   Remember that your partner doesn't define you. He's not your "other half" either. He compliments you, but he does not complete you.

Chapter Eight

Love the One You're With—You!

I don't think I've been able to look at myself naked since I had my first child five years ago. I just can't face looking at my stretch marks.

—AMELIA, AGE 37

I'm really happy spending time on my own. Sometimes, I enjoy my own company just as much as I enjoy being with my partner. Life's good.

—TARA, AGE 49

THE MOST IMPORTANT RELATIONSHIP in our lives is our relationship with ourselves. Loving yourself should be the starting place for all your relationships, not just your relationship with your partner. And to clarify further, it is the foundation for all healthy relationships. If you are currently feeling uncomfortable with the notion of loving yourself, then you need to explore the various ways

165

to change that. This means not just saying you love yourself on the surface of things, but making it really become true for you.

Now we could get really heavy and go all psychoanalytical on you, but we are here, after all, to talk about sex and making it hotter between you and your partner. What we have found is that when it comes to feeling both sexy and being sexual, a big part of that actually comes from you alone. It's not just about how you and your partner relate to one another, or what he says or does to get you hot. It's about you, how you feel about yourself, and the level of confidence you exude. This is where loving yourself comes into play.

For instance, how can your partner find you sexy if you don't? Even if you resemble Elle Macpherson in the nude, if you don't project the confidence that says "Yes, I'm sexy!" your partner isn't going to think so either. Think of your partner as a blank canvas, ready to receive you as whatever you're willing to project his way. We are what we feel, and what we feel is what we project to our intimate partner and to the world. Sexuality is not about having the perfect body, the most beautiful face, or the most expensive clothes or lingerie. None of that really matters. What does matter is how you feel about yourself. Sexuality comes from within, and that's why the way you feel about yourself has the most power of all.

Throughout the book we have stressed the importance of having a sexual dialogue with our partners. Well, this dialogue also includes our own inner dialogue with ourselves. You need to learn to love yourself first, and only then can a real, satisfying relationship with your partner flourish.

So . . . Let's Think About "Us" for a While!

How do you feel when you look in the mirror? Do you say to yourself, "Wow, I'm hot!" And if not, *why* not? Unfortunately, with all of the fashion and celebrity magazines that we look at every week—even if just while waiting in line at the grocery store—we have come to believe that unless you look twenty-five, weigh 120 pounds, and are 5'10", then forget it, you're just not that sexy. The amount of self-loathing women feel today is truly astounding, and it is ultimately so sad and pointless. We're all going to die one day. Do you really think you're going to look back at your life when you're ninety and think, *Wow, I'm so glad I was so critical of myself all those years.* We doubt it.

Besides, we know from personal experience how the photos in the magazines lie. Believe us, there is a lot of retouching going on! There is leg lengthening, figure reshaping, and of course the air-brushing of the wrinkles, zits, eye bags, blotchy skin, and, yes, cellulite. The skin in magazines is so heavily retouched nowadays, we wonder if there is any real skin left showing on those pages at all! So, stop thinking you have fallen short in any way. We all fall short of the perfection in magazines. Even the models themselves! They have been transformed into a pretty picture. An image. That's all. Let's fall in love with the reality of how wonderful we real women are for a change. That means each one of us embracing who we are in all our individual glory. Yes, zits, cellulite, wrinkles, and all!

Laura is a fifty-one-year-old personal trainer at a very upscale women's-only gym in Beverly Hills who specializes in training women over forty. She has a very engaging personality and an incredible love of life that attracts men and women alike. Her aerobics classes are always packed. Everyone loves Laura's energy, her big toothy smile, and the love she has for exercising. But Laura doesn't have a perfect figure. In fact, she's about fifteen pounds overweight. But that doesn't seem to affect her clientele's devotion or her husband's affection:

"I'm Italian, and I love to cook Italian dishes for my husband and my two daughters, so I know I'll probably never be skinny again like I was when I was thirty. But who cares? I know I can still be in shape and healthy and be a little overweight. In fact, my husband seems to like me even more these days because for the first time in my life I've got really good cleavage. When we go out, I like to wear low-cut dresses that emphasize my breasts, so I don't think anyone even notices my hips."

After talking with Laura for several hours, we realized that most of her personal-training clients, many of whom are considered Hollywood's most attractive women, are sadly unhappy with themselves and their sexuality.

"I have one client, an actress, who is only forty, but she has already had numerous plastic surgeries on her breasts, face, and body. The sad thing is that when I met her ten years ago, she looked so much better. She was about a size six—slim, but not too slim—and she looked like a normal healthy California girl. Now she's a size zero, and her face looks older than her age because it looks so false. It's almost like she could be any age, even sixty, but trying to look younger. And the cute butt she used to have years ago is gone, too. In fact, she told me she has to buy clothes sometimes in the children's department. She's *that* thin. When I ask her if she's happy with the way she looks, she always says, "God no! I've got some cellulite here, my boobs could be bigger, I need to plump up my lips some more, and I'm thinking about having labia surgery . . . " and on and on. She's never happy, no matter how many times she tries to change herself. She told me she hardly has sex with her husband anymore either. I think she's so unhappy with herself that she's just not in the mood. Her unhappiness and insecurity with herself shows, and that makes her even less attractive, too.

"I have other clients who are less overweight than me, but they refuse to look in the mirror at the gym, even with their gym clothes on! When I tell them it would really help with certain exercises to look in the mirror to check their form, they refuse. They say "Look, Laura, I'm not going to look in the mirror, so please just stand in front of it for me." I've never met so many insecure and unhappy women in my life, but I guess it's common. All the money and fame in the world can't buy self-esteem, I guess."

The Mirror Is Your Friend

The first place to start if you want to begin feeling sexy again is to look in the mirror. We know many of you may just run by the mirror every day after you get out of the shower and refuse to look at it, much like Laura's gym clients, but this has *got* to stop if you want to start having a great sex life again. Earlier, we explained the importance of looking at your partner every day. Well, it's also very important to take a good look at *yourself,* too.

Before you get dressed in the morning, when changing your clothes for an evening out, or even before you go to bed at night, take a moment or two to stand in front of the mirror. Naked. Yes, naked. Really look at yourself. Look at your breasts, your rear, your waist, your legs. You can even sit on a chair and look at your vagina if you like. Then say to yourself, "I'm sexy," and really mean it and feel it. Run your hands over your skin and the feel the lines of your body. Feel your shape, your breasts, and your rear. Feel your skin, how soft it is, all the while thinking to yourself, *I'm sexy, I'm fabulous, and I'm worthy.* Do this every day until it starts to ring true in your mind. Then after looking at your body for at least a couple of minutes, try on the sexiest pair of shoes that you have in your closet. Put them on and strut around the room (yep, still naked), and repeat to yourself while looking in the mirror, "I'm incredibly sexy." This may sound silly at first, but believe us, this is important. You need to get into the habit of looking at your body naked and loving it—whether you weigh 100 or 300 pounds, whether you're tall and lanky or short and curvy. Your body is beautiful and you've got to start realizing that and really believing it. Rejoice in your individuality and your uniqueness.

Many women don't like to look in the mirror "until they've lost a few pounds," but why wait for something that may or may not happen? Why wait to start loving yourself? This doesn't mean that you become self-centered, narcissistic, or arrogant about your appearance. It just means you start to embrace who you are—extra pounds, stretch marks, wrinkles, cellulite, and all. And once you love your body, it will be much easier for your partner to love it, too. The following story illustrates the power that the beauty of a woman's body can have once she accepts herself.

From a very young age, our friend Nikki has always been a little overweight. In fact, all the women in her family are overweight too. In high school she was a size ten, and by the time she was in her twenties she was a size sixteen—not obese, but certainly heavy. She had tried every diet under the sun—Weight Watchers, Jenny Craig, Nutrisystem, and more—but nothing seemed to work for her. She would lose thirty pounds and then gain back forty. She was always shy about showing her body, even though she has a very nicely proportioned hourglass figure with ample breasts, a round rear end, and shapely legs:

"Ever since my teenage years, I would hide my body because I thought I was so fat compared to my friends. When I got into the grunge music scene in my twenties, it suited my style because I could wear baggy shirts and big old jeans and continue to hide my shape. I never had many boyfriends—I think because I really didn't like my physical self very much. When I was in my early thirties, I wasn't wearing grunge-type stuff anymore, but I continued to wear loose clothing. I would even buy men's dress shirts and button them nearly to the top with baggy pants underneath. I work as a textbook editor, so it doesn't really matter what I wear to work because I don't have much contact with the public.

"One day recently though, after my last diet failure, I saw a big article in a magazine about this singer named Beth Ditto and noticed in the pictures that although she was even bigger than me, all the clothes she wore were really tight and sexy! To be honest, I was surprised at first that she had the guts to wear sexy stuff like that when she was probably a size eighteen. But she really did look sexy and great! Seeing her being hailed as this sexy goddess made me think about how I viewed myself. I mean, she seemed so confident and cool in those pictures. It was clear to me she just didn't care that she was big; she just embraced her larger-than-life size and all its glory.

"Because of her, I decided to turn over a new leaf and accept myself the way I was too. I mean, if she could do it, so could I! 'I don't need to be thin to look hot and be sexy,' I said to myself. It's not like I gorge myself anyway, and I eat pretty healthy too. Besides, my body is just naturally happier being this weight. And, it's not like there's this huge pot of gold on the other side of Thinville! 'My life is really good right now and so is my body,' I kept saying to myself.

"I dumped all of my baggy men's shirts and high-waisted baggy trousers, and started to shop for some clothes that might show off my body more. I bought a black cocktail dress and black stilettos as well—which made me look so much taller and thinner than I actually am. Believe it or not, I had never even bought high heels before! I also bought low-cut jeans, sexy tops that showed my cleavage, and some daytime dresses that hugged my waist. Nothing trashy—just casual, feminine, sexy clothes for daytime and evening. From there I was emboldened to get my hair cut, styled, and colored, and I tried wearing a little more makeup, too. I even got a pedicure for the first time in my life! It's like my very own makeover guardian angel shined down upon me and decided to give me a boost in the right direction.

"The first time I went out with my friends looking this way, their jaws dropped! They couldn't believe I was the same person. They all thought I had lost weight or had liposuction. It felt great because I did it just for myself and not for anyone else—I wanted to treat myself and be selfish for a change. Men started paying more attention to me as well. To be honest, it was a little scary to get so much attention at first, but I still loved every minute of it. And all this happened because I saw Beth Ditto and saw how sexy she was dressing! My life and image of myself have changed dramatically for the better because of it. And you know what? Now I can even look at myself naked in the mirror and say, 'Girl, you're hot!'"

Nikki is a very brave woman. It's very hard to look in the mirror and accept ourselves absolutely, without condition. But it's something we must learn to do to be truly happy and content with ourselves.

The Naked Truth

On the subject of looking at ourselves in the flesh, one of the things that really amazed us when we started doing research for this book was that no one ever suggested the obvious—that sleeping naked every night with your partner will increase your chances of having sex. Is it *that* simple? Yes, it's that simple. Going to bed every night with a flannel nightgown, socks, and underwear is yet another bad everyday habit that hurts your chances of being intimate with your partner. And the same goes for him. When he goes to bed with the same old T-shirt and torn underwear every night (c'mon it usually is torn, isn't it?), what does that say to you about how he feels toward you sexually? It doesn't make you feel sexually wanted, does it? What a surprise.

When we spoke to women for this book, one of the questions we always asked was "What do you and your husband wear to bed every night?" The women who said something like "I usually wear nothing except a little perfume," would almost always be happier with their sex lives than the women who said they wore night-clothes. Even the women who said they only wore underwear had less sex than women who didn't. Why is this, you ask? Because when you go to bed with clothes on, even if it's just underwear and a T-shirt, you are saying to your partner that you are not willing to be naked with him, and that carries a lot of implications. It means you don't want him to reach out and feel your naked waist, your soft breasts, and your warm thighs. It doesn't matter if you live in North Dakota in the winter—use another quilt for goodness' sake! Isn't your marriage and your own happiness worth it? Unless you're on your period or you feel sick, you should always climb into bed naked with your partner, and he should do the same. Wearing sexy lingerie is always fun—especially if it makes you feel sexy—but the key is to sleep naked more often than not. Sure, the latest teddy from Victoria's Secret could be worn once in a while to mix things up. But the standard attire should always be this: nothing.

We also found when we chatted to women about this subject, the ones who slept naked generally had a better body image and were more comfortable in their own skin than women who had to put on a nightgown before hopping into bed. We found that the women who slept naked weren't necessarily more gorgeous, younger, or thinner than the women who wore nightclothes. But the signal it sent to their partners is that they felt good about their bodies and they wanted to share them with the men they loved.

Also, once you start sleeping naked with your partner, he's more than likely going to follow your lead and start doing the same. Why? Because he's going to feel awkward hugging you in bed and feeling your soft skin when he's still wearing that old T-shirt and torn underwear. Sex is a dance, and when you take the lead and set the stage, so to speak, he will soon follow, and you'll be enjoying the feeling of skin-on-skin contact that may have been sorely missing in your life. Sex is physical. Sex is all about touching, looking, and feeling. So how are you going to explore that side of each other when you're separated by flannel?

Claire, a hairdresser, and Danny, a computer programmer, have been together for seventeen years and married for twelve. They have two young daughters, ages seven and ten. Except for some financial problems in the past (they sadly lost all of their savings after investing in tech stocks a few years ago), their life together has been very good. They are devoted to their daughters, have regained their financial security in recent years, and live in a comfortable house that they have meticulously restored. Claire explained to us one evening:

"When we lost all of our savings eight years ago, we were so stressed that I don't think Danny and I had sex for at least a year. We were so depressed and stunned that we barely had the energy to take care of the girls, let alone have anything left over for sex. In the beginning of our relationship, we always slept without clothes on. It would have never occurred to us to sleep with anything on. When the girls were young though, they would sometimes sleep with us or jump in bed with us in the morning, so we started to wear pajamas because they were always with us. And then when we lost our savings, we never felt like having sex, so wearing pajamas became a habit that we just never got out of. I mean, we would have sex now and then, but not very often at all. It wasn't good.

"Even after we recovered from our financial disaster, and the girls had gotten older and weren't cuddling with us anymore, our sex life still didn't improve. I guess it was because to have sex, I would have to go to bed not wearing my usual flannel nightgown and Danny would have to take off his pajamas. Once we started always wearing nightclothes, it became kind of awkward to take them off before coming to bed. If I felt like having sex, I would sometimes try to wear something sexier than a nightgown, but I would end up feeling kind of silly because it felt so strange to be exposing my body. It seemed like I was broadcasting 'I want to have sex tonight!' and it just felt awkward to be so obvious about what I wanted. I also think that I had completely stopped looking at myself naked, so I probably wasn't very confident either. Once I had the girls, my stomach never went back to being as tight as it was before, and I know I have quite a bit of cellulite now too, so I wouldn't want to look at myself anymore, let alone have him look at me with the lights on before we got in bed.

"Anyway, one morning I caught myself in the mirror while I was wearing my nightgown buttoned up to the top, and I thought to myself, *My God, I look just like my mother, and she's sixty-eight! What's happened to me?* I really did miss the old days when Danny and I would sleep wearing nothing because when we did have sex, it just seemed so natural and easy. There was no 'broadcasting' going on beforehand. We would just start kissing and go from there. We both felt pretty hot for each other back then, so covering up didn't seem practical.

"So, one day I suggested to Danny that we should start sleeping naked together again. At first he was surprised and not that into it, but he decided to try it all the same. And after a while, it became our usual way of going to bed again. Now we not only have more sex, but the sex is better. It seems more spontaneous and more organic, and definitely more erotic. Recently, I spread my legs in bed while facing opposite him and let Danny get a good look at my vagina. Believe it or not, I don't think I ever had the confidence to let him look at me so intimately before. And the lights were on too, which is something I'd never done. It was like he was in a trance! I started touching my breasts and then my pussy. It was one of the more erotic moments in our sexual life together. When we got together, we were both kind of shy about sex, and even though we slept naked together back then, neither one of us had the confidence to really show our bodies in the most intimate way. After a few minutes of just staring at me, Danny finally said, 'God you're sexy. I can't wait to fuck you.' It was so cool! He'd never talked to me like that before, and it was so sexy to hear.

"I think the fact that I was feeling sexy about myself really turned him on the most. Now we take the time to look at each other in the light and really experience our bodies together. It's like I'm seeing him as a whole new man again, and I think he sees me as a truly sexual woman for the first time. I'm more turned on by our sex life now than I was even in the beginning of our marriage. Now that we're older and more confident and mature, I can't wait to see what will happen in the future! I think we're both finally uncovering our sexual selves—and it all started with just having the confidence to get naked again."

What we have found after talking to women like Claire is that when you wear clothes to bed every night, you make the chances of having sex that much harder. Do you really want to continue doing that? All Claire and Danny did was get naked before they went to bed, and then they upped the ante by really looking at one another in the light. The hard part for Claire was finding the confidence to feel great about her body. But, she overcame her fears and embraced herself for who she is *now*. And that's what made her so sexy—her confidence in herself.

Sadly, we have met many women who do not love and believe in themselves, and they desperately try to stay young and slim by exercising obsessively or by having plastic surgery. They do this with the futile hope that it will keep their partners from straying. However, being critical of your looks and constantly trying to improve yourself— like the woman at Laura's gym who is a size zero—only leads to more self-loathing and concentrating on what is *wrong* with your figure. Focus on what is wonderful about you, and love who you are now, not who you wish you were. There is only one you, and you need to project that to your partner and to the world. Enjoy the ride of being you. The real you.

You Are Luscious!

Imagine sinking your teeth into a big, fat, juicy cool peach on a hot summer day. Just imagine yourself doing that, with the juice running down your fingers and your chin. You lick your fingers because it tastes so good. You're slurping away, gobbling it up, and you don't have a care in the world except thinking about that luscious, sticky peach. It's really all about the peach, isn't it?

Well, your approach to your sexuality is like eating that luscious peach! You aren't thinking about how you are "performing" the task of eating that peach. You are just doing it and loving every second of it! When you look at your body in the mirror, think about the wonderfulness that your body is capable of. Think about your body as a luscious peach that is ripe and juicy and desired.

You can do so many amazing things with your body. Your body performs for you. When you look at yourself in this way, doesn't that make it easier to love yourself? We think so. Our bodies are the physical celebration of who we are. Why *not* celebrate that? After all, we do have only one body. If anything, it's never our body that is the problem anyway. Quite often, our problems are all in our head. This is why we want you to think of your sexuality like you are that peach (or any other messy sticky fruit that you adore), because you are gorgeous, luscious, juicy, and ripe for the plucking! The act of eating that fruit gets you out of your head and into the moment. If you are spending too much time thinking about how your body appears and how you are performing with your partner, you're staying way too much in your head. How are you going to enjoy the moment? How are you going to allow your body to just "get on with it" when your mind is in the way of all that? You certainly aren't going to be able to have an orgasm in that state of mind. So let yourself go. Be abandoned!

Don't Fake It, Baby

Speaking of orgasms, unfortunately many women still think of their partner's pleasure as being paramount to their own—probably because they don't allow themselves to get out of their own heads and into the moment. So, how many women have faked it? We can safely say that nearly all of the women we spoke to have done this sometime in their lives. Sometimes they do it just to get sex over with. Or sometimes, they just didn't want to hurt their partner's feelings. And sometimes it was because they wanted their partner to feel good about himself. Whatever the reason, they were way too much in their own heads and didn't allow their own bodies to enjoy themselves.

Obviously there are exceptions to this, and in one case, we spoke to a woman who was on an antidepressant drug for five years and was unable to achieve orgasm as a result. Antidepressants commonly cause this side effect, and if you take them, you need to tell your partner, so you can stop feeling guilty or bad. It's the drug and not you. In this particular instance, instead of this woman being honest with her husband, she decided to fake it. For five years! She was too afraid to hurt his feelings, even though the reason she couldn't reach orgasm was because of the drug and had nothing to do with him. But each time she faked it over the years, lying to herself and her husband, she got more and more into her head—filling it with guilt and remorse. With that kind of baggage going on there, how was she ever going to have an orgasm? The woman recently shared with us that she has since gone off the antidepressant, and guess what? She's still not able to have an orgasm. After all those years of faking it, even though the drug was gone, nothing changed. This is such a shame. She needs to be honest and open with herself and her partner, and get rid of all that baggage in her head. And all this went on because she wanted to please him.

Be Selfish!

We know it's hard to lay the "real thing" on a man and allow yourself the time to have an orgasm, especially if you're afraid to be totally honest. Often, we would rather just fake it to make them feel good, instead of actually really feeling good ourselves. But what is the sense in that? We all like to feel pleasure. Sure, we've heard the age-old saying that sex is about giving as well as receiving. Receiving in that respect means being a little selfish at times. Both partners need to have a level of selfishness and self-awareness in order to be truly giving to their mate. Where is the intimacy and the intensity of making love if you are so concerned with your partner and his needs that you ignore your own needs? And let's be honest, girls, men love it when they feel like they've done a good job! If you allow yourself to feel good, he'll feel even better.

In our last chapter we showed that maintaining a bit of separation from your partner is good for your relationship. Taking the time for yourself to explore who you are, your interests, and also your sexual needs means being a little selfish. And that selfishness originates from loving yourself. The following poignant story of a woman who failed to be selfish is all too common.

Beth and Cameron had been married for eighteen years until they divorced because Cameron had an affair and fell in love with a woman at work. Beth was so devastated that she had a nervous breakdown. After two years of therapy, she is finally able to talk about it:

"I thought Cameron and I had a great partnership. We both love our three kids, and we always spent all of our free time together. But I guess our sex life wasn't that great. I really thought that was normal after being together for almost twenty years. What I learned in therapy, which was a very painful process, was that I didn't help our sex life by faking it all those years. I had faked it with every man in my life, even my first high-school boyfriend. I think I was always too uptight to really enjoy sex, and I also thought that the man's pleasure was the main focus, so I ignored my own needs. It's not that I never got turned on, it's just that I never reached orgasm. Sometimes I would secretly masturbate after sex because I was turned on, and I had to have an orgasm to fall asleep.

"Anyway, after Cameron left, I had a string of one-night stands and short-term boyfriends, and even with them I would fake it! Can you believe it? I would fake it with a one-night stand—someone I would never see again and didn't even care about. I guess it's just a hard habit to break. Not that it's my fault that Cameron had an affair, but I do think that if I had been more selfish and thought about my own needs in bed, our sex life would have been more intimate and more interesting. I don't think he ever suspected, but I think that our bond would have been much closer if I had been honest. Also, because I never had an orgasm with him, my enthusiasm for sex wasn't that great, so I'm sure he picked up on that and maybe that's why he strayed."

What Beth's story so painfully illustrates is that when we think we're being selfless and pleasing the man, we are actually doing more harm to the relationship than we realize. When we always try to please our man and go along with his desires while ignoring our own, we are seriously damaging the relationship. Men pick up on when we are enthusiastic about sex. But, how can we be enthusiastic about something that gives us no pleasure? So make sure that you enjoy yourself in bed.

Of course, you need to know what pleases you sexually. If that is something you aren't quite sure about, then let discovering it be a time of fun and exploration with your partner. Your man will be thrilled at your pleasure and want to give you more of it. Every man loves to please a woman, so make sure you really are happy in bed. Give yourself that pleasure. Give your man that pleasure. Be brave, and lay the real thing on him!

So far in this chapter, we have been focusing mainly on loving and getting to know your physical self. But it should go without saying that truly loving and accepting your physical self means also knowing and loving your emotional and mental self—your inner self. Of course we aren't perfect. We all have our faults. But learning to love *all* of yourself in spite of those faults is key. Imperfections are what make you you! Revel and rejoice in that. Perfect can be boring.

Knowing yourself—your skills, talents, tastes, and mind—will attract the kind of man that you would want to attract. And, hopefully, if you have enough love and respect for yourself to start with, you will know that you've attracted the right partner in the first place.

However, when it comes to long-term relationships, we can sometimes lose our way in knowing and loving ourselves. We can become so engulfed in the relationship that we lose that sense of self and all the confidence that goes with it. And yes, all those years of calling each other "honey" and "pookie" and "Mommy" and "Daddy" can certainly take their toll on how you feel about yourself.

This is why our previous chapter on separation is so important. When you explore who you are as an individual, it allows you to continually learn about yourself, and your tastes, talents, and strengths. This gives you a positive outlook, reinforces the love and respect you should have for yourself, and keeps your confidence level up. Loving yourself means always being on that quest to discover all the aspects of who you are. It means continually improving and excelling in those things that excite you and utilizing those aspects of yourself that make you unique and wonderful.

When you're happy with yourself, your partner will pick up on it. This will fuel his desire for you and his desire for more sex, and vice versa. Sexuality is contagious between partners. When you have the confidence to really believe that both your inner and outer self are special and should be celebrated, you will find yourself celebrating with your partner. When both partners are happy and fulfilled as individuals, the frisson between them amplifies many times over. Your sexuality will always find a way to grow if you allow it. If it's living, evolving, and maturing, it will keep *all* aspects of your lives together exciting—not just the sexual aspect.

Throughout our book, we have talked about the habits and behaviors that you need to change to have a more fulfilling sex life. Sometimes, having little or no sex is just the easiest road to take. Unfortunately, it's not the right road. In our society, long-term relationships are not seen as the haven for hot sex that they can be. Most couples feel almost embarrassed if their sex life is great. And if it isn't, they feel that's normal and languish in their own un-happiness—because you know what they say, "Everyone's sex life is like this after a while."

Additionally, many people cringe when they think of couples in long-term relationships having sex, especially if they're over fifty. Why? What is wrong with our silly society in that respect? As we age, we learn *more* about ourselves—we know more of who we are and what "floats our boat." Sex is often portrayed as something only for the young in new relationships. But let's think back and ponder that one for a bit. Sure, you may have been horny and excited, but wasn't it sometimes awkward? You were probably both more enthusiastic than accomplished at lovemaking. Your partner didn't really know you and you didn't really know your partner. You may have had your clothes off, but you weren't really naked. Truly naked.

But sex with someone whom you truly know, love, and understand—sex with someone you have a past with, someone you have a future with, and someone who is your true life-partner—that's the deep-est, most pleasurable, and hottest sex of all. Sex with a long-term partner is one of the truly magical experiences we are offered on this earth. It can transcend us, it can transform us, and it can take us to a world of love and pleasure like no other. This kind of sex is one of the greatest rewards of a long-term relationship.

In the end, this book hasn't been just about rekindling your sexual selves with your partner. It's really about exploring all the parts of yourself that are valuable and unique. As women and men, we are many things: wife/husband/partner, mother/father, career person, homemaker, cook, housekeeper, gardener, caregiver for humans and animals alike, philanthropist, dreamer, believer, doer. All of the things that we are—and can be—should be embraced in this life. So, we aren't *just* talking about sex. Sure, sex is fun. Sometimes it's dirty, raunchy, and hot. And sometimes, sex is truly about being intimate—a way of expressing deep love for your partner. Sex is all of these things at different times. As much as we have had such fun writing and doing research for this book, we feel that we have a very important message, too, a deep message: We must embrace all aspects of ourselves. We must explore and embrace our potential—mentally, emotionally, and physically. We need to be empowered by all the good things our bodies and minds are capable of. All of these aspects of our humanity make us whole. If we deny ourselves sex with our loved one, we are also denying a very integral part of ourselves. We have this one life to live—let's live it fully and completely.

LOVING YOURSELF

1 Focus on the wonderful things that are uniquely you, and stop obsessing about your so-called faults. Embrace the image you see in the mirror today, and stop focusing on tomorrow.

2 Be confident in your own nakedness and always sleep naked with your partner.

3 Treat your sexuality like a luscious peach—devour it with abandon. Let your body take over, and give your mind a rest.

4 Be selfish and be truthful. Stop trying to please each other at the risk of not pleasing yourself. Being selfish can save your relationship, while being overly selfless can ruin the truthfulness and intimacy between you.

5 Love the inner core of who you are and constantly explore and nurture your true spirit. When you truly love yourself, your most exciting sexual and life experiences lie in front of you.

Epilogue:
The Ten Couple Commandments

WE'VE CREATED THESE TEN COUPLE COMMANDMENTS so you can easily review some of the main concepts in this book. Take a few moments every now and then and revisit them. They will help to refresh your memory and to keep you renewing that important bond with your partner . . . again . . . and again . . . and again!!!

1   I will relish and enjoy calling my partner by his/her own name.

2   I will never call my partner "honey," "sweetie," or any other silly pet name.

3   I will never use baby talk, baby-type voices, or call my partner "Mommy" or "Daddy."

4   I will always give my partner privacy and respect when it comes to all things having to do with the bathroom and bodily functions.

5 I will always find the time each day to look into my partner's eyes and let the silence between us rekindle our desire.

6 I will always remember to use touch and body language to express my desire for my partner.

7 I will speak to my partner like a sexual adult, and not be afraid to talk a little dirty sometimes.

8 I will rejoice in our difference of opinions, and yes, argue about them!

9 I will always maintain a separate identity from my role in the relationship, and be passionate about my own life, as well as encouraging my partner's separate identity.

10 I will love and accept myself the way I am today—mentally, emotionally, and physically—and I will encourage my partner to do the same.

We hope you enjoyed reading our book, and have found valuable advice in it that you can incorporate into your daily life. We wrote this book for all of us—so that we can all have happy, fulfilling lives, and, of course, great sex!

For more advice, information, and updates, please go to our website: www.stopcallinghimhoney.com.

Index